What Others Are Saying . . .

"*Eureka!* has opened the portal to the next level of rehabilitation—a level only the caregiver with intimate knowledge of the patient can provide. When the professionals had reached the limits of their skills, this used to be seen as the most that could be accomplished. No longer!"

Lawrence J. Beuret, M.D.

"As a Certified Therapeutic Recreational Specialist on an acute physical rehabilitation unit for 24 years, I would want every person who suddenly becomes a caregiver to a person with a traumatic brain injury to read this book. The use of the subconscious was a key to Eve's rehabilitation. By aligning her subconscious suggestions with the patient's lifelong beliefs, needs and values, the author has really gone from a caregiver to a rehabilitator. We need more such creative rehabilitation ideas with realistic expectations."

Ben Johnson, M.S., C.T.R.S.

"As a Public Health Professional, I highly recommend this book to all caretakers—especially those caring for brain-injured patients. *Eureka!* not only gives caretakers specific techniques to deal with very difficult and intensive situations, it provides invaluable information on how to take care of the caretaker in the process. It gives readers inspiration and concrete tools to help in their daily lives."

Rhonda Kolberg, R.N., B.S.N., M.S.

"In my work with stroke and brain injury survivors and their families over the years, I have come to believe that recovery is truly a "we are doing this together" proposition for both patient and caregiver. When stroke or tbi strike, it is not just the patient who has to deal with the consequences. The caregiver is equally involved—and maybe more so, since many patients are unaware of all the effects of the "disability." Caregiving is a 24 hour job. Sooner or later, the caregiver learns that taking care of his or her own needs is of utmost importance. If the caregiver is ill and can't do the job, who is going to do it? *Eureka!* certainly brings a refreshing approach, in which the patient and caregiver learn together how to have a good time, while dealing with what is quite often, a devastating loss."

Sharon Prosser, B.S.W., C.S.W. Case-Worker, Green Bay WI

"*Eureka!* highlights how vital the caregiver's personal health of mind, body and emotion is to the monumental task of leading the stroke/brain trauma patient up the mountain of discouragement to seemingly impossible heights. With her characteristic conversational style and self-deprecating humor, Madonna Siles makes this book another of her page-turners. As a lay person, she tells what she has found out through self-knowledge, experience, pluck and creative efforts. Any who have brain-damaged patients in their care will find this book fascinating, as well as challenging and cause for hope. How little we really know about the human brain, and how much this book teaches us to believe in what persevering care can bring about."

Suzanne Zuercher, O.S.B.; Licensed Clinical Psychologist; Author of *Enneagram Spirituality* and *Enneagram Companions*

Eureka!
Memories and Motivations

A Strategy for Creating
a Healing Home for
the Stroke/Brain Injury
Patient and Caregiver

Madonna Siles, C.P.C.

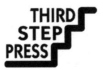

Cover art and interior design by Kathryn Marcellino, MarcellinoDesign.com
Illustrations by Madonna Siles

Third Step Press
520 N. 7th Avenue
Sturgeon Bay, WI 54235
e-mail: tsp@eurekamaster.com
www.eurekamaster.com

Quantity discounts are available to your company, institution or organization. For more information, contact the publisher at the address or e-mail above.

Publisher's Cataloging-in-Publication

Siles, Madonna.
    Eureka! : memories and motivations : a strategy for
creating a healing home for the stroke/brain injury
patient and caregiver / Madonna Siles.
        p. cm.
        LCCN 2009936860
        ISBN-13: 978-0-9825518-0-6
        ISBN-10: 0-9825518-0-0

    1. Cerebrovascular disease--Patients--Rehabilitation.
    2. Cerebrovascular disease--Patients--Biography.
    3. Aneurysms--Patients--Rehabilitation. 4. Aneurysms--
    Patients--Biography. 5. Brain--Wounds and injuries--
    Alternative treatment. 6. Caregivers. 7. Caregivers--
    Biography.   I. Title.

RC388.5.S495 2010
362.196'81'00922
                QBI09-600165

                ISBN-13: 978-0-9825518-0-6

Dedicated to the Eureka! Memory-Makers in My Life

Cheery Chrissy, whose wit and wise insights
brighten the days; good friend Merle, who
never ceases to surprise and delight;
artists Karsten and Ellen, whose vibrant
visions of Door County decorate my life;
and unforgettable Mom

Contents

Acknowledgements

This book evolved with the support and encouragement of my cheerleaders: Peggy Savides, Christine Shults and Dana Kasprzyk. I am grateful for the expert help of my editors extraordinaire: Kevin Beuret, a poet and writer in his own right, and Marilyn (you are the best) Johnson, who deleted my ellipses with a flourish. A special thank you to my talented and patient book designer, Kathryn Marcellino.

Eureka! was inspired by the memory-makers in Eve's life and mine. Thank you: Merle Ketelsen, Anthony Costanza, Bruce Shivley, Dr. Tom and Eileen Phelan, Karsten and Ellen Topelmann, Fran Holdren, Karen Piwowarski, Fran Corn, Ron and Penny Latko, Jim Smith, Simone Brumleve, Suzanne Zuercher, Thea Jarvis, Jean Handel-Bailey, Cathy Causby, Paul Savides, Kathy White, Gloria Muczynski, Suzyn Mills, Max Ots, M.D., Sharon Prosser, Julie Feld, M.S.W., Tracy Bielinski, R.N., Mary Vietzke, R.N., Norm and Doris Henning, Jim and Jennifer Berns, Susan Powers, R.N., Nancy Stults, R.N., Sue Crass, Mary Claire McHugh, Laurie Thiede, Kathleen and Nora Finnerty, Joel Herrick, Helen Anschutz, Nancy Uttech, Marge Grutzmacher, Nikki Welch, M.D., Deborah Fleck, Jan Lockhart, Rick Okie, Christa Braschnewitz, Candy Borkowicz, Fran Elliot, Fannie Tsang, Mary Rowles, Richard Williams, and Lawrence Beuret, M.D.

We also wish to acknowledge our spiritual support group which includes our Higher Powers and these angels in heaven: Valerie

Samuelson, Roger Ketelsen, Patricia Moeller, Richard Kasprzyk, Arlene Smith, Ginny Frohman, Johnny and Zosia Patka, Harry "Grampy" Brumleve, Steve and Mary Siles. Thank you for being there day and night.

I must acknowledge one more angel who guided me through this book. Dr. Gordon E. White, University of Illinois, was not only my creative advertising instructor many years ago; he was a friend and mentor, too. I will never forget his inspiring stories about the great ad campaigns from the glory days of advertising. Dr. White was a legendary copywriter, author and Eureka! teacher.

This book could never have been written without Yolanda and friends, who showed me how to be happy, joyous and free—one day at a time.

Foreword

You may be paging through this book hoping it is the how-to manual you are searching for: How to fix a brain-injured person. This book *is* about caregiving brain-injured patients, but not in the way you might think. As you'll soon see, it is about you and your own brain which, as it turns out, is your best asset for being a good caregiver.

In 1987 I needed this book, but it hadn't been written yet. I was sitting in the waiting room of our hospital's intensive care unit, waiting for my next opportunity to sit with my eight-year-old daughter. She was in a coma, unconscious with a head injury, after being hit by a car as she waited for the school bus.

I was a registered nurse in a different unit at the same hospital, but none of my experience or training prepared me for my role as a brain-injury rehabilitator. I felt like I was just a mother, and that it wasn't enough.

What Madonna Siles shows in her book is that our relationships *are* enough, but again, not quite the way you might think.

Eve and Madonna were close friends. But after a few months of caregiving, Madonna found herself examining her own side of it. She realized she had to start taking care of herself in order to be relaxed enough to read the cues Eve was giving her, to use her intuition to perceive Eve's needs. Madonna also discovered that when she was the most relaxed she had her best, most creative ideas. In the relaxed frame of mind, the ordinary events of day-to-day living became opportunities for brain healing.

Professionals in rehab services refer to mental skills such as organizing, prioritizing and sequencing. I remember wondering where I might find such a workbook for my daughter.

I was missing the obvious: The opportunities to practice those mental skills abounded in ordinary life. Something as simple as going out for a few hours involved choosing appropriate clothes (warm or light jacket), planning an agenda (visit Grandma, go to the library, go to the grocery store) and bringing needed items (school art to show Grandma, library books to return, grocery list). Eureka! A pleasant afternoon becomes a brain-healing experience.

Madonna's background is advertising, where she learned that emotion is a powerful link to memory. She knew that practicing mental skills workbook-style can be painfully dull. But by adding emotion, whether it was spontaneous and silly or deeply heart-warming, Madonna made those tasks interesting, so the memories would *stick*. I know her accounts have *stuck* in my mind. What could have been a series of stories weighted with guilt or sadness has become memorable, thanks to Madonna's quick application of humor. As she points out, humor is one of the most powerful emotion-evoking tools we caregivers have readily available.

No matter what your relationship is to the patient, helping a brain-injured person recover demands your very best. Madonna has drawn the best from herself, her education and her experience and used it creatively in Eve's recovery from brain injury. Her book is the story of the process she used and how you can apply it to your caregiving situation.

Peggy Savides, R.N.

Introduction

They said I should pull the plug on my comatose friend, Eve, after her level-five brain aneurysm.

They said my minimally functional friend had come as far as she was going to after six months of hospitalization and rehabilitation.

They said there was only a two-year window for significant brain recovery.

They said there was little I could do. I should just wait and see.

They were wrong. There was something I could do. After the insurance ran out—and professional rehabilitation became an unaffordable luxury—I tried to become a home-schooled expert on brain repair and rehabilitation. But every time I found a book or website that I thought might help, it contained a warning that every stroke/brain injury was different; so I should consult our physician. I was back to square one.

Eventually I realized I had two choices: run away or stay and try to figure out a way to help Eve. I decided to try—one day at a time. Over the next few months I transformed myself from a clueless caregiver into a brain rehabilitator, and created a home healing environment where Eve's brain could be encouraged to heal itself. Perhaps, more importantly, I discovered that the key to our healing strategy was for me to take care of my needs, my motivations, and my health first. To my surprise, what sounded selfish on the surface was actually the smartest strategy for our survival.

Six years ago, Eve smashed through the two-year window of

recovery, and she has been significantly improving ever since. This year she will be 65. Talk about myths and miracles.

Did the heavens intervene? I certainly hope so; I prayed enough. But truly, I believe most of the miracles happened to me as I slowly learned to be a patient, imaginative and intuitive caregiver.

In order to save Eve and myself, I created Eureka!—an emotion-based, motivational strategy for recovering and restoring both the caregiver's and the patient's mind/body/spirit. Every day, we are getting better together.

This Eureka! strategy evolved over time. I knew something was working when I realized Eve was continually and significantly improving long after the two-year deadline for stroke recovery. Will my approach work for all stroke and traumatic brain injury situations? Honestly, I don't know. But common sense suggests it offers possibilities.

For sure, my approach is not very scientific by today's medical standards. But what good are scientific studies and significant statistics if they aren't translated into practical techniques for home caregivers?

I truly wanted the medical professionals to tell me how to do it. If only one medical/rehabilitation professional had taken the time to teach me to become an emotion-based, motivational therapist at home, I could have saved a lot of time and devoted more energy to the healing process. Instead, I had to learn what is in this book from my experience with Eve, one day at a time.

Emotions are such powerful brain rehabilitation tools. The most powerful ones can be found in the patient-home caregiver emotional healing connection. Perhaps the medical/rehabilitation community is not properly "motivated" to explore the use of emotions as a viable home-healing strategy for brains. Creating an emotion-based strategy is time-consuming; and as we all know, time is money.

Well, I had the motivation and I had the time—24 hours a day, seven days a week. Surprisingly enough, I also had the expertise. I had been creating emotion-based, persuasive appeals to motivate action all my life in my career as an advertising writer and creative visualizer.

Now on with the story of how my Eureka! strategy developed and how I customized it to work for Eve and me. You'll find many ideas and suggestions on how you can customize Eureka! for your caregiving situation. Most importantly, you'll find ideas on how to become more intuitive, stress-free and emotionally motivated on a daily basis.

Hopefully, you'll learn, as I have, that "brain" caregiving is a challenging, intriguing and inspirational journey. In other words, what I thought originally was a colossal problem has turned into a heavenly gift and an opportunity to explore and become the "me" I always wanted to be.

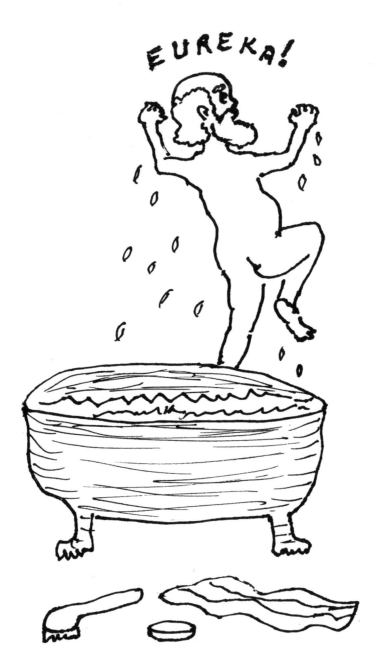

1

Inspiration for the Eureka! Strategy

Way back when I was a little kid, I read a book about the scientists whose discoveries changed mankind's way of doing things. Of all the stories, my favorite was the one about Archimedes.

As the story goes, Archimedes was about to take a bath when he made his amazing discovery. As he lowered his body into the tub, he caused the water level to rise. It clicked in his brain: water displacement—what an ingenious way to measure the purity of gold. "Eureka!" he exclaimed. "I have found it." Then, according to my imagination, the stark naked Archimedes jumped up, ran out the door, and raced down the street, shouting "Eureka!" to surprised passers-by.

What fun! I decided to become a scientist when I grew up. After failing a high school chemistry test, I changed my mind.

No matter. By then I had realized what really intrigued me about the Archimedes story was the action of creating that memorable "Eureka!" moment. And so I studied the art and science of persuasive communications. I became an advertising copywriter, where my job was to create memorable "Eureka!" moments to persuade the public to take action and buy my clients' products.

Little did I know that this ability to create enthusiastic, high-impact, emotional Eureka! moments, messages and memories would someday serve me in persuading my best friend, Eve, to recover from devastating brain damage. At age 56, she was the miraculous survivor of a near-fatal brain aneurysm. It wreaked havoc with her mind, body and spirit. When she finally came home after months of hospitalization and rehabilitation, Eve was the shell of a functioning human being.

I promised God, the angels and anyone else who would listen to do my best as a caregiver, if they would help me bring back the "old Eve."

And so they did, by sending me the idea for Eureka!

The Eureka! strategy takes advantage of the powerful emotional bond between home caregiver and patient. With Eureka! that emotional bond becomes the major motivator for a better, healthier, more successful life for both the patient and the caregiver.

Who cares about the caregiver's health? Well, I did. And once you realize how the health of the caregiver's mind, body and spirit can absolutely, positively influence the patient's rehabilitation and recovery, you might care about the caregiver, too.

Very quickly, I realized that I could do nothing for Eve unless I took care of myself—whether I wanted to or not. First, I had to get my own body, mind and spirit in shape by controlling stress—one day at a time. I had to practice relaxing every day—no matter how ludicrous that concept seemed—with crises swirling around me. I had to learn to walk through each day with no expectations for Eve's recovery, but great expectations for me. I had to accept my powerlessness over Eve's recovery before I could start building a home environment to encourage Eve's brain to heal itself. As I wrote in my first book, *Brain, Heal Thyself*, I had to learn to trust my own intuition in lieu of the medical professional help I desperately wanted, but could not afford or was otherwise not available.

Once I was in shape I could begin implementing the Eureka! strategy with the patient. The Eureka! emotion-based strategy is a complement to traditional therapies (speech, physical, cognitive, occupational). It doesn't replace any prescribed medical courses of action; it can enhance them.

I never wanted to develop my own home-caregiving strategy. Nope; I figured the medical profession owed Eve that. Her recovery had cost her dearly. She came home with a few instructions—but not enough to keep her going beyond a barely functioning level. Certainly, modern medicine had saved Eve's life, but had left her without any way to live it.

So I tried to help her. Because I tried, I believe the heavens blessed me with a way to create a successful, healing home environment for both of us—the Eureka! daily living strategy.

Throughout this book I explain how Eureka! worked for us. Then I offer suggestions on how to adapt what we did to create your own unique Eureka! recovery strategy. Hopefully, both of you will experience the success and creative rewards Eureka! has brought to Eve and to me.

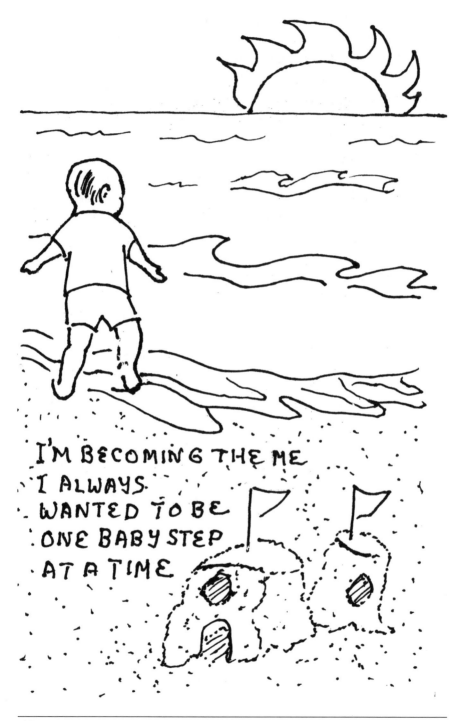

2

Preview of Eureka!

"Wait two years and then see what you've got," the neurosurgeon said. I nodded, held my hand out to my brain-damaged friend and led her out his office door, muttering to myself all the way down the hall.

The neurosurgeon and I first met on the night 56 year-old Eve had arrived at the Green Bay hospital by ambulance. She was the doubtful survivor of a level-five brain aneurysm. She was rushed into brain surgery—not the usual practice for brain aneurysm victims—but in this case it was necessary to save her life. That night the neurosurgeon and I had discussed her chances. I said to him, "No extraordinary measures."

He said, "Eve is young. She deserves a chance, right?" He neglected to tell me that the odds against her full recovery were monumental. He said she would probably be more subdued and less communicative. Looking at Eve now, as we slowly exited the hospital, I would have selected different words to describe the possible outcome. "Blob" or "zombie" might have been more appropriate.

After months of hospitalization and rehab, Eve had finally come home. She did not come with any "instructions," except that I should invest in an over-the-door pulley weight system to exercise her frozen shoulder. Oh, yes, they also told me to make her work logic puzzles and fill out a daily journal. Eve did not want to do any of this. To this day, I have a complete collection of every style of 2002 daily calendars. They are all in pristine condition.

Looking back, I realized I had blown my chance to escape from the hopeless caregiving situation that now faced me. When Eve was still in the first hospital, a social worker had advised me to empty the bank account, then run as far and as fast as I could. That's how dismal Eve's future appeared to be. Unfortunately, I was old enough to know that running away was not the solution for my problems. I had learned that no matter where you go, you bring yourself along. I didn't have very many positive personality traits; but loyalty was one of them. Eve and I had committed to taking care of each other if one of us got sick. If I had known about brain aneurysms then, I might have moved to strike that from our pact. But I didn't know. To make matters worse for my wiggly will, I did know that if the situation was reversed, Eve would never abandon me.

In my first book, *Brain, Heal Thyself*, I describe how I developed my seat-of-the-pants caregiver strategy. As a matter of fact, that strategy is still evolving today. It has two equally important aims: to bring back the mind, body and spirit of my good friend Eve, and to preserve my health, sanity and serenity in the process. Frankly, I never, ever wanted to create my own brain-healing strategy. But the medical community of doctors and therapists (though well-intentioned) gave me so very little to go on for home caregiving. I had to fill the days with something. I was a 24/7 caregiver anyway and their minimal directions took no time at all.

What I never expected was that my strategy would do anything, except hopefully give me a reason to wake up every morning. I couldn't afford to fool myself (or anybody else) that love of my friend Eve was my primary motivation. Self-preservation in the midst of crisis was my goal. In the end, I believe that self-honesty saved us both.

How my "brain, heal thyself" strategy came to be is described in my first book. Here, in this book, I describe how my Eureka! strategy evolved, what worked for us and what didn't over the next eight years. Although I believe a caregiver's presence is still required for Eve to survive 24/7, most of my days belong to me— and hers to her. Happily, the "old" Eve has come back, complete with her character flaws and foibles, as well as her engaging personality and sense of humor. That's all I ever asked of her, of me, and of the heavens.

The ideas in this book are simple, easy and cost little to implement. The hard part was to convince myself to follow a daily relaxation program, so that I could relax on self-command in the face of frustration and crises. After a few run-ins with the consequences of stress, I decided it was worth my time to follow my own relaxation program.

In addition, I outline the importance of coming to terms with reality, boosting a belief system, recognizing caregiver motivations as well as the patient's, and implementing routines punctuated with creative challenges and enthusiastic adventures.

That's what I did. I was grateful that it kept me sane and serene. But I was amazed at how well it worked for Eve. Who could have guessed that taking care of myself as a caregiver would be so important to my friend's brain rehabilitation?

In this book, we'll discuss the theoretical powers of the amazing subconscious mind. I'll explain its various roles as the protector of the patient's survival, the storage center for memories, and the keeper of belief and value systems—the source of motivation. I'll also discuss how the relaxed state helps caregivers stay in touch with their own emotions, motivations and needs. As a bonus, we'll see how a truly relaxed state enables two-way communication with a patient who won't or can't talk, or who confabulates, or who doesn't make much sense at all.

As the book progresses, I'll put all of this together in an approach to memory making and retrieval that can be uniquely adapted to many caregiving situations. We'll discover how the simple tools and gimmicks used in advertising products can easily be adapted to brain rehabilitation situations. Spurred by enthusiasm, this emotional and creative approach to everyday living works on many levels. It's a "We will get better together" team approach that can transform an ordinary day into a rehabilitation opportunity for the patient and a rewarding experience for the caregiver.

As the old adage says, a picture is worth a thousand words. Even though I'm a writer by trade, I couldn't agree more. That's why you'll find pictures at the end of this book. Actually, I call them motivational meditation billboards.

Just like the billboards we see along the highway, these billboards are designed to evoke emotional responses. Not gushy feelings, but emotions that motivate. If they accomplish that, then they have a good chance of being remembered—not forever, but occasionally throughout the day.

We'll also make use of the power of advertising to make an indelible impression on the subconscious mind. No, we won't be selling products. For our rehab purposes, we will be exploring the quirky way powerful ads of the past are linked to memories of what we were doing, saying or feeling in the heyday of the commercial.

For example, almost any beer commercial triggers my childhood memory of a comical, beer-bellied cartoon bear who danced to the beat of tom-toms. Not only can I recall the jingle; I'm also instantly transported back 50 years ago to our family room where Dad watched the Sunday afternoon baseball game on TV. The memory is so vivid that I can feel the summer breeze blowing through the window and smell the aroma of Mom's Sunday supper emanating from the kitchen.

This powerful mechanism—this ability to bring back yesterday's memories with all the emotional trimmings and connections to physical and cognitive memories—is what I call Eureka! It's the basis for the strategy I used for Eve's brain rehabilitation and recovery.

The success of Eureka! on any given day depends on a variety of techniques and attitudes that are relatively easy for the caregiver to master. We'll discuss all of them in the coming chapters.

Ultimately, you'll see how easy it is to create your own simple yet powerful motivational messages to inspire recovery in the patient and more rewards for the caregiver.

Before I begin explaining all the elements of Eureka! I thought I would emphasize again my belief, based on my experience, that if caregivers do not take care of themselves while dealing with brain damage, they will be of little help to the patient. Having support is very important to the process. If you haven't gathered your support network yet, please start tomorrow. For today and tonight, maybe this story will help.

Many years ago, when I was still a beginner in the 12-Step program, I found myself floundering on one dark and lonely night. My latest sponsor, in a succession of sponsors, had resigned. I guess I wasn't very teachable. However, I was desperate. Reluctantly I dialed the phone number of the only woman I could think of to help me. She was a tough one, known for her "no nonsense" style of A.A. sponsorship.

"Will you be my sponsor?" I asked her timidly, trembling at the thought.

"No," she quickly replied. "I have too many people to sponsor."

I whimpered into the phone.

"Okay, okay, don't whine." She continued, "I will sponsor you temporarily. What's the problem?"

"I'm scared," I said. "I don't know what I'm supposed to do, except go to meetings. It's midnight. There are no meetings."

"Okay, calm down," she said quietly. "Now I'm going to recite a prayer to you. Write it down. 'Lord, help me see what I have to see, hear what I have to hear, say what I have to say, do what I have to do, in order to do Your will today.' Got it? Okay. Then wash your face and get ready for bed. Think about the prayer until you fall asleep. Call me tomorrow morning and tell me what it means to you."

I thanked her and hung up. I started to cry. I was so grateful that somebody had finally given me something concrete to do. I repeated that prayer until I fell into blissful sleep. Twenty-two years later that woman is still my "temporary" sponsor.

In the 12-Step tradition of "Pass it on," I'm suggesting you find your support amongst your friends and relatives. Until then, you can post on my website (Eurekamaster.com), which I monitor every day.

SUGGESTION:

Just in case you're feeling as desperate now as I was then, here's a suggestion for you:

1. Take three deep breaths.
2. Recite a little prayer or just ask for help from the sun or the stars above. Then call a friend and ask him or her to please lend you an ear for a few minutes. Tell your friend how you are feeling. Ask if they can suggest an action for you to take.
3. Afterward, you can choose to do the action your friend suggested—or not. If not, then you can do this one. I suggest you clean a window. You'll know why when you are finished. No matter which action you take, you should feel better than you did before. If not, do another action (preferably a boring one), until you are tired enough to fall asleep.

3

The Brain Aneurysm that Devastated Both Patient and Caregiver

On an incredibly beautiful, but otherwise ordinary, Indian summer day in 2001, my friend and housemate, Eve, was weeding the yard. Suddenly her head exploded in pain. The pain was so intense that it knocked her to the ground, like a lightening bolt out of the blue. Meanwhile I was inside the house when I heard the moans. Frantically, I raced around, searching for the source. Could it be a wounded animal trapped under our porch?

No, it was Eve, crawling into the living room, collapsing in a thrashing heap, holding her head and moaning. I called 911, not sure if Eve had a migraine headache, not knowing she was in heart failure. The paramedics came and rushed Eve away to the county hospital, leaving me standing in the kitchen—clueless as to what was wrong with Eve. It was a state of mind I'd be in for many months to follow.

By early evening Eve had been transported to the northeast Wisconsin regional brain trauma center at a Green Bay hospital. She had a grand mal seizure in the ambulance. The seizure sent her to the doorstep of the pearly gates. The neurosurgeon recommended immediate life-saving surgery to repair the devastation caused by the exploding brain aneurysm. I reluctantly agreed. (We had reciprocal legal powers of attorney papers that explicitly stated "no extraordinary measures" for either of us.)

Little did I know how extraordinary this surgery was, as was the one she had two days later (to bring her back from clinical death). Following that surgery, Eve went into a coma. Within a week she experienced brain-frying seizures that prompted the doctors to put her in a deeper drug-induced coma to save her brain. As the neurologist explained, "If we don't do this, her brain will be completely 'fried' in a few days."

Apparently, the insurance company didn't want to waste all that money on a patient who was virtually a cognitive "vegetable." After 30 days, they ordered comatose Eve out of the hospital and into a nursing home. Like most insurance policies, Eve's provided less than two weeks of nursing home coverage. Convincing a nursing home to admit a patient without Medicaid coverage was a bit of a challenge. But I found one willing to take a chance on Eve—and me. It was privately-owned, with a warm, caring staff, from the top nurse to everyday aides. A month later, Eve emerged from her coma, and walked with a walker. She couldn't speak; her swallowing apparatus was paralyzed. At that point, the neurosurgeon promised that a shunt-implant would help. It did, and Eve could talk again by Christmas, though much of what she said didn't make sense.

Meanwhile, I, the caregiver, was feeling the stress effects of an almost daily four-hour round trip drive to Green Bay. I couldn't eat, my back hurt and my teeth ached. I had my own "brain" challenges, not that anyone particularly cared. I was depressed by our rapidly dwindling finances, the fear of the mortgage coming due, and the onslaught of medical bills that fell into two calendar year deductible periods. Plus, there was a statistically improbable array of bills for procedures that cost more than the "usual and customary" charges, per the insurance company. But more about my problems later.

Back to Eve. It was month four of recovery and we were on the road—a five-hour trip to Chicago for Eve's one-month stay in a reputable rehabilitation hospital. The best I could say about the experience was that it made it easier for Eve's lifelong friends to visit her. That camaraderie was of utmost importance for her continued recovery. As for the "professional" rehabilitation aspect, well, the lack of concerned attention certainly contributed to the undoing of the continence training Eve had received in the nursing home.

Eve walked into the rehab hospital by herself. When the rehab month was done, they wanted to send her home with a wheelchair. Duh. However, they did teach her how to balance a checkbook (the presumption being that she had money in the bank) and they taught me the gyrations I would need to accomplish a shower for two. Lord, how I dreaded that.

And then Eve came home. Lucky for us, the insurance company had worked out a deal with northeast Wisconsin's brain rehabilitation center for Eve to receive physical, occupational, speech, cognitive and psychological therapy three full days a week. I was so happy to be "home" in small-town Wisconsin, where the staff treated patients and caregivers like human beings.

On our days off from the outpatient process, it was just Eve and me and a few caring Chicago friends who telephoned frequently. Naturally, they wanted to talk to Eve when they called. Eve's conversations sounded flat and emotionless. When she got off the phone, she had no idea who had been on the other end of the line. And even a hint from me, such as the friend's first name, didn't inspire any recognition in her eyes. Eve was a zombie. I was scared.

After several weeks of staring into her vacant eyes, I began to panic. Was this my role for the rest of my life—caregiving an empty shell who bore no resemblance to my friend? Now I did want to run away; but it was too late, too complicated. Our money was tied up in the house and our not-yet-open art gallery. And always, there was the knowing that if the situation was reversed, Eve would not abandon me. Sadly, I was very aware that I wasn't just a clueless caregiver; I was a coward, too. My new reality overwhelmed me— physically, mentally and emotionally.

As the three months of therapy was drawing to a close, I decided it was time for me to get real and start dealing with life on life's terms.

Reality—such an over-rated concept on TV—is certainly nothing I desired in my everyday life. I'm a big fan of dreams, wishes, fairytale endings and miracles. At first glance, the reality of Eve's situation was that she was still a long way from functioning. Here's what I wrote in my journal.

"Eve walks into walls, so there's a problem somewhere in her balance system—her vision, inner ear or in the messages sent to or from her brain. Nobody can tell me where. Her ability to sense her bodily needs is defective. She goes to the bathroom by the clock, rather than per the urge. She is oblivious to changes in her body temperature. Her right side is weakened. Her swallowing mechanism is also weakened. She still has a feeding tube protruding from her tummy.

"Mentally, she can't perceive problems, so obviously she can't come up with solutions, let alone choose the best one. She suffers from long-term memory loss and her short-term memory is spotty. She can't comprehend the concept of future, so planning is out of the question. She is able to read, but is indiscriminate in her choices, and seems to prefer cereal boxes over books. She retains little. I can't hold her attention in a conversation for very long; she spaces out after a couple of minutes. I'm not sure if she comprehends all that I tell her. I know she doesn't invite conversations. When she does talk, she confabulates to fill in blanks. She often says her deceased mom or dad visited her today. She thinks our two pet cats are my dogs.

"Emotionally—now this is weird—she laughs and smiles too much and often inappropriately. She says she's happy; but she's never sad or fearful. I suspect that her answer to "Are you happy?" should more exactly be "I'm comfortable." She can't remember what makes one old friend different from another. Very few moments in our everyday life spark any emotional reaction at all."

I forced myself to write this list of Eve's disabilities rationally, so that I could get a grasp on our reality. I had no idea what the cure was for anything or if a cure even existed. I knew the professional rehabilitators were focusing on freeing up her frozen shoulder and strengthening her weakened right side. Though Eve was able to solve logic puzzles in speech therapy, she was resistant to keeping a daily calendar. The therapist didn't like this; so she "fired" Eve (as if Eve was resisting on purpose?). Eve was "lost" in the cognitive therapy class on problem-solving, but she said it was her favorite session. Last, but not least, Eve had found her calling as the world's best vacuumer in occupational therapy. This was encouraging, if not too practical. At home we had hardwood floors.

The time had come for Eve's insurance-appointed graduation from outpatient therapy. I was reminded by the staff that Eve had a two-year window for recovery and there was nothing more I could do to help her along.

For the sake of my sanity, I couldn't afford to accept this. So every day I led Eve on a two-block walk to the post office. She zigzagged all the way, but arrived back home still standing. It gave me hope that a miracle would happen before the therapy insurance coverage ended for the year.

On Eve's last day of therapy, my hopes were dashed. At her final meeting, the staff gave me some shoulder exercises for Eve and instructions to continue playing word games and "Keep on vacuuming." As Eve careened down the hall, one staff member patted my shoulder and said what everyone was thinking. "We're sorry, but we believe Eve has come as far as she's going to."

From that point on, any further recovery and rehabilitation was up to me.

4

Breaking through the Two-Year Window for Significant Recovery

My previous book, *Brain, Heal Thyself*, highlights the first two years of Eve's recovery. I actually wrote that book over a year later; but I didn't include the third year. It wasn't that Eve didn't improve; she did. In truth, I simply could not quantitatively describe it. Nor could I effectively explain what she or I did to cause the many little "leaps" into a higher-functioning level.

Yes, anyone could see that Eve had broken through the two-year window for significant recovery. It's taken all of these years of observation for me to understand how my homemade caregiving activities could have contributed to Eve's breakthrough. I admit my experiments were not very scientific—and I left the door wide open for any miracles God wanted to send our way. What I do know is that none of our activities hindered the healing process.

As I said, the activities were not very scientific. Most of them were not repeatable or measurable. How many times could anyone find the first spring wildflower peeking through the snow? Frame a painting for our gallery? Pack boxes for moving to a new home? Or celebrate the 4th of July? However, as time went on, I realized all of these Eureka! activities shared common attributes: They were all laced with high-impact, memory-making, emotional appeal.

Yes, I intuitively believe these Eureka! activities led to the leaps in Eve's recovery. Fortunately for both of us, I continued to create more and more of them, without the blessing of science. I wasn't sure why; I trusted I knew how. I was operating by the seat of my pants—practicing at-home brain recovery based on intuition. I now know what a blessing it was to not know what I was doing, scientifically speaking. If I had, I would never have given myself permission to be creative, inject spur-of-the-moment enthusiasm, over-the-top emotion and intuition into my quest to bring back Eve's body, mind and spirit.

It was not logical to do what I did with Eve. If I had listened to the scientific opinions of the doctors, if I had truly believed there would be no significant recovery after two years, I would have handed Eve the TV remote and let her entertain herself for the rest of her life.

Instead, I continued to push and pull her through the days. I developed a hodge-podge home caregiving program that utilized concepts from the 12-Step program's team teaching approach and shamelessly borrowed from Dale Carnegie's enthusiastic approach to basic public speaking. I also used Emmett Fox's sermons on non-resistance and "letting go" of expectations and turning over solutions of problems to God.

I also relied on an eclectic combination of emotional motivation and persuasion techniques gleaned from my lifetime career as an advertising copywriter. And I never doubted my scientifically unproven belief about the amazing capabilities and motivational power of the subconscious mind, much of which I had learned from my friend, Lawrence J. Beuret, M.D. I proceeded to create the Eureka! strategy based on the unfounded assumption that the brain aneurysm had not damaged Eve's subconscious (wherever it was). I acted on that assumption relentlessly by teaming my subconscious with hers in a daily effort to persuade Eve's broken brain to heal itself.

What's amazing to me is that all of this worked for Eve's recovery, despite the simple fact that I placed my needs first. Life and my experience with the 12-Step program had taught me that if I wasn't okay, I would never be able to help Eve.

That certainly sounds like a very selfish approach to caregiving. No wonder it's taken me so many years to muster the courage to write this book. But today, I can confidently say my strategy worked for us. As you will see, I believe it could help most every home caregiver of a cognitively, emotionally challenged stroke or brain injury patient, if the caregiver takes the time to customize this approach to his or her situation.

5

Resist Not Relaxing

Why do we caregivers resist relaxing? This question has dogged me ever since Eve's brain aneurysm eight years ago. After all, I know how important relaxation is. Perhaps part of the problem is that relaxing while in the middle of a caregiving crisis (or in any continuously frustrating situation) is really hard work.

I can still recall bristling with irritation when the neurosurgeon told me that he didn't know if Eve would ever emerge from the coma. Then, two minutes later, he told me to go home and relax.

Of all the choices I had for activities when I returned home, relaxing on purpose was at the bottom of my list. The thought was ludicrous. After all, I had phone calls to make, dishes to wash, clothes to launder, cats to feed.

But what did I do when I arrived at home? I popped open a can of diet soda, grabbed a handful of potato chips, and plopped down at the dining table. Then I proceeded to stare out the kitchen window for the next half-hour, while I munched empty calories and fed my depression. In the end, all I accomplished was to feel very sorry for myself, for Eve, and our desperate, dismal life situation.

When I finally roused myself from the table, I felt guilty about the unfinished housework. Naturally, I plunged into my chores, promising myself I could take a relaxation break in two hours when I made my phone calls. Excuse me. Since when is delivering bad news to friends and family an opportunity to relax? But I had already wasted a half-hour on self-pity.

And that was okay. Not too smart—not very healthy—but considering the bad news, it was understandable. However, it didn't make any sense at all to punish and fool myself by pretending that those dreaded phone calls would be relaxing. I had to make myself understand that there was a difference between purposefully relaxing body, mind and spirit and the nonphysical activities I mistakenly considered relaxing. Really, truly, there is nothing relaxing about the boring four-hour round trip drive to Green Bay—the emotional phone updates for friends—or sitting at the table wondering what I should or could do next. All of it was exhausting.

On the other hand, I knew that purposefully pausing to savor a cup of herbal tea and soak my tired body in a tub of bubbles was relaxing. My problem was my resistance to planning my days well enough to inject a regular relaxation break. Obviously, I wasn't in enough pain (physically and emotionally) to set aside time at the start and finish of each day to calm my body, mind and spirit. This was a choice. It didn't take long for me to pay a price for letting stress run unchecked in my daily life.

One morning I couldn't get out of bed. Somehow, some way, I had hurt my back. It took me three days to get going again. Meanwhile, nobody had visited Eve in the hospital. This convinced me to begin a relaxation program. I started off the next day, reading a short meditation followed by a calming walk around the backyard. At night, I sipped a ritual cup of tea, followed by a soothing, sleep-inducing bubble bath. It worked. I was very relaxed for about four days. But on the fifth morning, I bolted from the house without taking my walk. According to my schedule, I was late for the hospital, even though no one was expecting me, let alone comatose Eve. Feeling guilty, I took an extra-long bath that night. On day six, I skipped my morning relaxation routine again. And that night I was simply too tired to take a bath. By day seven, the whole relaxation concept had unraveled.

Not surprisingly, my feelings of being overwhelmed returned. My back was hurting again and now I was grinding my teeth in my sleep. Ouch! I had to take my precious free time and make an appointment at the dentist.

Why did I let this happen? I can think of lots of reasons, but I'll focus on these. All are convoluted, but maybe you'll be able to relate.

First, let's look at day four of my aborted relaxation program. In the morning, I noticed that I was feeling pretty good on my drive to the hospital and during my visit with Eve. I was still feeling okay on the drive home. I was relaxed. Suddenly, the thought hit me that I didn't deserve to feel relaxed or good, considering Eve's condition. I couldn't shake the thought. So now the stage was set for my self-sabotage.

I took a poll of the voices in my head. "How dare you feel relaxed?" they said. "You don't deserve a moment's rest while Eve is sick."

Honestly, who would ever say that to me? Eve's friends and distant family? Not likely. My friends? I doubt it. The crowd of faceless people in my mind—those judgmental onlookers who have defined the qualities that make up the perfect caregiver? Bingo.

According to the movie in my mind, all perfect caregivers are constantly, unselfishly concerned with the well-being of the patient. Personal sacrifice is the ideal, preferably with a smile on one's face. If the caregiver has a few moments to feel good, that time would be better spent thinking up even more good deeds to benefit the patient.

Oh, heck, I'm already a failure. I am having a hard time just psyching myself to travel two hours to the hospital to stare at a comatose patient for an hour. Meanwhile, I'm failing on the administration side of the coin, too. Every day I reorganize the pile of bills I don't know how to pay; then I reread an insurance policy I can't comprehend, and I try to logically plan for a future that seems as mysterious and scary as any horror movie. Therefore, I conclude, I have no right to feel relaxed.

Was that really my thought process? I'm afraid so. Now, I don't presume most people sabotage their own well-being to this extent. But I'll bet there are other caregivers that can relate to the following excuse (er, reason) for not managing their stress.

Now, don't laugh. I've actually entertained this thought, too. If I, the primary caregiver, appear to be calm and in control, nobody is going to bother to call or visit. I'll bet there's even a caregiver or two who might worry that no one will help them with caregiving tasks or household chores unless the caregiver appears to be on the verge of panic.

Never does it occur to me that I could simply ask for my friends' help and support or call in a favor or two. Better to whine than be looked upon as a less-than-perfect caregiver. Anyway, folks expect a good caregiver to show a little stress. It's part of the role.

I believe all these mental gyrations emanate from the nebulous nature of brain caregiving. Unlike end-of-life caregiving, the brain caregiver is often required to vacillate from a compassionate, sympathetic approach to a tough-love stance. No one seems willing to offer a prognosis for recovery or a rehabilitation plan to get there. But everyone agrees there is reason to hope for recovery. That hope puts unrelenting pressure on the caregiver.

In other words, the message to the stroke or brain-trauma caregiver unfortunately appears to be: If you pray the right prayer, dance the correct dance, you too might someday have a functioning patient again. So you begin each new day facing a foggy future of not knowing whether anything you do will have any affect on the patient.

The day will be frustrating, filled with miscommunications, and in the end the patient probably won't be able to thank you for your patience. And yet, there are many situations where the stroke and brain trauma patients recover various functions—spontaneously, relatively quickly or very, very slowly. So there's hope. And where there's hope, there's the stress of knowing that something you, the caregiver, can do will make a difference.

What happens if you are one of those few rare caregivers who simply can't relax, no matter how hard you try?

That's easy. Quit trying. But first let me tell you a true story. This incident took place over 20 years ago.

One night I was riding in the car, coming home from a 12-Step program meeting with my sponsor. She was driving; I was moping. Though I had managed to string together three months of sobriety, I was exhausted and depressed. I had done everything I was told to do—daily meetings, constant prayer, counseling, socializing with strangers. As far as I could see, nothing worked. There was no joy in sobriety for me. I was jobless, penniless, friendless and despairing.

"I don't think I'll last another week," I said aloud as we drove along. I scooted closer to the car door, not sure what my sponsor's reaction would be to this sudden burst of honesty.

She kept both hands on the steering wheel as she turned to look at me. I searched her eyes for empathy, sympathy—even pity would have been nice. Instead, her usually light blue eyes were dark and smoldering. Uh-oh.

Quickly, I responded to the threat. I didn't want to make her mad at me. I said, "You know I've followed all the rules. I've tried to work the "steps." I've done what you've told me to do. But nothing's happened. I don't feel any better. I crave a drink every minute of the day. I'm scared I'll lose my mind if I drink again; but this 12-Step program doesn't work for me. What more could I do?" I moaned.

My sponsor shifted in her seat; the car swerved slightly. I saw her fist coming at me. I winced, but her fist flew past my chin into the dashboard.

"! & * ! x !," she sputtered like a volcano, ready to erupt. I was trembling. She continued, "Don't you get it yet?" She wasn't yelling; she was pleading. "Stop fighting it. You're gonna win. Surrender to the process. Don't you know you've got to con yourself into sobriety?"

A light went on, illuminating my dim, dull, soggy brain. I get it! Really I do. She was right. If I keep fighting myself, I will most certainly win. No matter that the prize is a wretched existence or slow agonizing death: I'll win it.

"I think I finally understand," I muttered meekly.

"Good," she said, as she pulled into the driveway. "God willing, I'll see you tomorrow. Meanwhile, don't forget the short version of the first three "steps": "I can't; He can; let Him.""

Back to now. If I was your relaxation "sponsor," would we be having a similar discussion about your resistance to taking time out to care for yourself?

If so, may I suggest a self-con to save your life? Try asking the heavens for the willingness to try relaxing. That's easy, isn't it?

6

For Fast Relief

This chapter is for those caregivers who don't know or practice a daily program of physical/mental/emotional relaxation for the body, mind and spirit.

There are oodles of relaxation aids and methods available to all of us. I have friends who swear that flickering candles and aromatic oils do the trick for them. Others practice yoga or tai chi, go for a swim, or chant "ummmm." A lucky few can afford facials, massages, cruises and vacations to tropical isles. (Unfortunately, just thinking about the latter brings me dangerously close to jealousy—an emotion I cannot afford to entertain.) Anyway, there are plenty of vicarious vacations I can take in my imagination, if I just invest a little time and effort.

All of the aforementioned techniques are great. Mine, on the other hand, are much simpler. Before we start discussing them, let's take a deep breath, hold it, count to three, and exhale very, very slowly. We'll do that twice again.

How does that feel? I'll bet my three breaths were more relaxing than yours, and I'll tell you why. It's not that I've been given a special talent or gift from the gods. My ability to achieve a relaxed state quickly and easily comes from practicing it.

Fear not. Anyone can do it. If you commit to trying to relax ten minutes each morning, noon and night for 21 days, you'll be amazed at how quickly it will happen for you by day 22. (Mark your calendars now!)

To save time, we're going to multitask by including several mind and spirit relaxation exercises that can be done at the same time as the simple physical exercises. Note: As with any exercise program, it's a good idea to clear the exercise with a medical professional.

Now back to this fast, fast, fast approach to total relaxation in 21 days.

Here's how this easy holistic approach unfolds for me on any given day. In the morning, while I am munching cereal or drinking my coffee, I read an inspirational message from one of my favorite books. Sometimes it's the Bible, or a 12-Step program meditation book. It can also be a thought for the day from a website, such as mine. I often say a prayer, too, but always in combination with a meditation message. I want to give my brain something positive to think about during the day. Then I go for a walk—around the house or down the block. Even if it's January in Wisconsin, I want to let my senses get in touch with the day and the great outdoors. I take three deep breaths of the chilly air. Don't ask me why. Somehow it helps. Maybe it reminds me of my place in the natural unfolding of another day in a very big universe. Then I take three deep breaths again. I'm off and running. On with the day!

Around noon, I relax after lunch. Sometimes I sit in a quiet room at home and close my eyes for ten minutes. Or I sit in my car, put the seat back and close my eyes and breathe. I enjoy day-dreaming about my favorite beach scenes and woodland wildflower paths. Or if I'm motivated, I take another teeny-tiny walk. After three deep breaths, I'm rejuvenated. No afternoon slump for me.

At night, I usually give myself a wind-down signal a half-hour before bedtime. I microwave a cup of herbal tea and sip it while watching the TV. (I rarely watch the late night news. There are too many disturbing happenings in this world that are totally beyond my control. It simply makes me feel sad.) On the nights I feel sore or sorry for myself, I treat myself to a warm, soothing bubble bath.

Not only does it make me feel calmer, it's a good way to get clean (multitasking at its best).

There's more to do before bed, including one of the most dramatic, life-changing self-help techniques I have ever practiced. I call it the five-minute gratitude-with-a-twist list.

Being grateful is a way of life in the 12-Step program. Early on, many folks strongly suggested I write a nightly gratitude list. I tried it. B-O-R-I-N-G. At least my list was. How many ways can you say thank you for my job, my cat, my car, my food, clothing and shelter? Yes, I was thankful I had these things. Yet, the list didn't inspire me. What I really, really wanted back then—and now—was to feel as though God and the angels gave a whit whether I lived or died. Then as now, I was alone (except for Eve, of course). I wanted someone to hug me, even if it was only in my mind.

So I created a variation on the daily gratitude list. I decided to include the aforementioned food and shelter gifts. I didn't want the heavens to think I was ungrateful and take them away. The twist I added focused on all those good things that happened to me during the day over which I had no influence or control. I called those happenings miracles. (So does the dictionary.) My daily gratitude-with-a-twist list included anything good that I wasn't planning for or expecting.

Initially, I set my standards very low for determining events and happenings worthy of my miracle list. For example, if I was exiting Walmart laden with packages and a young teenaged boy held open the door for me, then that was a miracle. If someone treated me to coffee and a hot fudge sundae after a 12-Step meeting, that was another miracle. Unexpected paying jobs, checks in the mail, a helpful clerk, a phone call from a caring friend, a free car wash, a sale on Twinkies, you name it. If it was unexpected, and not the result of my manipulations, it made the list.

The first night I tried it, I aimed for three such mini-miracles. In five minutes I had listed five, on a day I would have previously labeled "okay, but not great." Day after day, month after month, there never was a night I didn't have something for my list. One item was rare; five items were the average.

I was simply amazed. I hadn't realized my trouble-ridden life was so very good. Obviously, somebody "up there" did care. For that I was grateful indeed.

After the gratitude list, I had one more trick before I attempted to count myself to sleep. I imagined grabbing all those really hairy problems in my head and locking them up in the jewelry case on my dresser for overnight safekeeping. I figured they'd all be there in the morning and maybe the elves, or God, or even my subconscious mind might solve them overnight.

Be very forgiving of yourself if you fall down while trying to learn to become more relaxed. It's nigh impossible to learn a new technique if you're feeling anxious. Hopefully, the anxiety is not a constant state, so that you can grab a minute or two to practice deep breathing and/or have a chance to close your eyes and daydream about a faraway peaceful place. If you really, really look for them, you'll discover more relaxation opportunities during the day—eyes of the storm—where you can practice a relaxation technique or two.

If you do nothing else, practice the progressive relaxation technique while trying to fall asleep. It beats counting sheep. (Since they all look alike, I frequently lose track of where I am and have to start over.) This simple technique has whisked me to dreamland on nights nothing else could help.

Before we begin progressive relaxation, say your prayers. Seriously. If bedtime is prayer time for you, then pray before you begin the routine. (Don't forget to pray for help in relaxing.) Chances are you'll be sound asleep before you finish it. By the way, here's an insight on the power of prayer that I learned when I joined the 12-Step program. Normally, I would never dream of telling anyone else how to pray, but this might help you as it helped me.

I was surprised to learn that the way I always prayed was setting me up for frustration, disappointment and, potentially, anger. Who wants to do that? Quite frankly, many of my lifelong prayers sounded as if I was a kid sitting on Santa Claus's lap: "Dear God, please—don't let me get fired—please make Mom well."

The reality was I didn't get along with the boss, so I was going to get the axe, and my mother had raging cancer for which there was no cure. I have no way of knowing what is best for me or another person.

I'm not saying I couldn't hope for a miracle or ask for one. However, my spiritual psyche would have been much better served by a prayer that also included, "Please give me the strength to handle the outcome—good or bad. Help me to learn what I have to learn and show me how to find the good and hopeful in what now seems to be such an unhappy situation."

I don't know if changing my prayers made them any more powerful, but I felt better after saying them this way.

Now, on to progressive relaxation. The room is dark, the house is quiet, and the patient is already sleeping. To begin, I silently ask my subconscious mind to let me sleep through the night and awaken me only in case there is a real emergency.

Then I begin: On the count of one, breathing in, holding that breath, 1-2-3-4-5. On the count of two, exhaling slowly. On the count of three, breathing in, holding that breath, 1-2-3-4-5. On the count of four, exhaling slowly. On the count of five, breathing in, holding that breath, 1-2-3-4-5. On the count of six, exhaling slowly. Etc, etc. All the way to the count of twenty.

If I'm still awake (often I'm not), I can begin progressive relaxation, using the imaginary feeling of warm, glowing, softly swirling energy to soothe aching muscles, tired old bones, and sluggish circulation.

Here's what I say to myself: Feel the relaxation begin in your toes, massaging your feet, ankles, legs, thighs. The relaxation progresses around your butt and into your lower back where it kneads, and swirls, and soothes, until you feel the tension begin to go. Moving on, the energy spreads out over your back and comes together at your shoulders, massaging the muscles until they begin to let go of tension. And now the energy travels down your arms, into your hands and fingers. You can move your fingers if you want to, releasing any and all tightness. Then slowly the energy goes back up your arms, revisits those shoulders, and enters your neck area. Now you pause while the energy caresses those muscles, pressing slightly as the tenseness is released, soothing away any pain or discomfort brought on by the day.

When it's done, the energy continues on, into the face muscles, unclenching teeth, massaging the jaw, caressing the cheeks and soothing your furrowed brow. Finally, it enters your head where it whisks away worries and calms your mind.

If I can still concentrate, I focus my thoughts on colors or clouds or endless ocean waves, but usually I'm gone.

For many years, I relied on relaxation tapes. There are many such CDs available on websites, including mine. Over the years I've learned to trust my own thoughts more. So, during the winter I play one of those nature CDs with new age music combined with the sounds of waves while I progressively relax. During the summer, nothing is more soothing to me than the sound of chirping crickets outside my wide-open bedroom window. Over the years, I've discovered that even weird rhythmic noises can lull me to sleep: the low rumble of truck traffic, the far-off whistle of a train, and even nightly coyote howling (but not until I had lived in Arizona for several years). To each his own; you'll soon discover your own technique.

7

Mumbo-Jumbo

After learning how to relax for a few days, I began training my body and mind to relax on command. Whenever I felt the need or urge to relax, I took three deep breaths and said my key phrase: "Now is the time."

I made relaxing a habit every day. Each morning I gave myself a suggestion, after reading my daily meditation, to "breathe" three times during the day. In the beginning, my results were spotty. Sometimes I could feel the relaxation; sometimes nothing seemed to happen. Nevertheless, I kept trying.

In earlier years, this learned skill helped me survive numerous dentist appointments for too many root canals. In a relaxed state, I could replace fear with quiet calm and distract myself from feeling any pain. On the job, it increased my ability to focus so that I could write faster. It allowed me to make creative connections, even under the pressure of a looming deadline. In client meetings, I replaced fear with focus. I learned to listen better.

After Eve's aneurysm, I used the technique to cope with care-giving stress, frustration and fear. I also used it before I began any creative thinking projects. It became a tool to help me figure out ways to handle finances, memorize meetings with doctors, and tune into Eve's needs.

As time went on I used relaxation as the base for recognizing rehabilitation opportunities in everyday life. In other words, the ability to relax on self-command became the magic key that opened the door to the subconscious mind where memories and creative strategies awaited discovery.

Whoa! Wait a second. Isn't the subconscious mind a bunch of mumbo-jumbo?

Perhaps. It hasn't yet been proven if or where it exists, although certain "powers" usually attributed to the subconscious mind are the subjects of scientific studies. Other attributes of the subconscious mind have gone from theory into practice and are being proved in the field.

For example, there are many athletes who report amazing results from regularly visualizing throwing a ball, swinging a bat, putting a golf ball, to increase their proficiency in a sport. Wi-Fi gaming for stroke or brain trauma rehabilitation is an expensive variation on this theme. Bringing that concept closer to home, Eve imagined she was successfully driving the car from the passenger seat for months before she ever took the wheel. This simple technique utilizes the subconscious mind's ability to "remember" imagined successes as if they are real. It's called "acting as-if."

But there are other equally powerful aspects of subconscious mind performance that could also be harnessed for caregiving application.

Here are two more attributes of the subconscious mind that I believed in and employed for home caregiving. I believed the subconscious is the storehouse for long-term memory (since birth). I also believed the subconscious mind is the keeper and protector of an individual's value and belief system.

There is no doubt that both of these functions happen somewhere in the mind/body. Subconscious mind advocates believe that they are not independent functions. They theorize that the memory keeping and motivation systems are linked. That theorized link is what I used to build my Eureka! recovery strategy for Eve and me. This link is an emotional—not logical—connection. It connects the past to the present and to the person's belief (motivation) system.

Here's how that link might play out in my everyday life. This is a very simple example of a powerful connection. Incidentally, I'm using potato chips for this example. Feel free to be imaginative and substitute your memory of candy, a teddy bear or cookies and milk.

Let's imagine it's the end of an ordinary, but stressful, workday. I return home from work and head straight for the pantry. I feel hungry—but what do I want to eat? Logically, I know it's time for dinner. Should I bring out all the good makings for a nutritional dinner? Instead I head straight for the bag of potato chips. Of course, my logical, conscious mind warns me that this is not the time to indulge in empty calories. Once I start, I won't stop eating them. I'll ruin my dinner. Do I listen to logic or do I grab the chips and head for the cushy sofa and my TV remote? You know me too well by now.

Why am I doing this? Why does my willpower pale in the face of a flimsy potato chip? Truth is that iron will and logical arguments don't stand a chance against my emotion-based belief that potato chips will make me feel safe, loved and appreciated. (In addition, they're a tasty treat.)

How can a little chip cause me to feel all those emotions? (By the way, the physical feeling is faint; it's the emotions that are powerful.)

With my first nibble of the crunchy, salty chips, I travel back in time. I am not consciously aware I am doing this. But on a subconscious level, I am revisiting my first potato chip memory, circa the age of six. It doesn't matter if I actually consciously recall the memory. (In my case, it just so happens that I can remember it as if it was yesterday.) It's important to realize that even without conscious awareness, my initial potato chip memory will be "touched" by today and reinforced by today's experience because the feelings are similar.

Here's how this past-present link unfolds. Pay close attention to the details I relate. Most have nothing to do with potato chips, but have everything to do with my emotional state back then—and now. As I recall, I was about six years old. It was a Saturday night. I was fresh from my bubble bath, dressed in my snuggly warm flannel PJ's with the floppy feet and yellow bunny rabbit design. As my little brother and I waited to hear the chime of the doorbell, the TV was playing "champagne music" from The Lawrence Welk Show. It was past my bedtime, and certainly past my younger brother's. (Life can be so unfair.)

It was the first time we had permission to stay up late to greet the guests for Mommy and Daddy's grownup party. Soon the guests arrived. Mostly relatives, they filed into the kitchen to hug and kiss my brother and me as we sat at the table with our shiny red little bowls of potato chips and our juice glasses brimming with soda pop, another special treat. Mommy had said I would feel sleepy by the time I finished my potato chips. She was right. Soon I toddled off to bed feeling loved, warm, safe and happy. As I drifted off to dreamland, I could still hear Lawrence Welk's band playing in the background.

Why is the memory so powerful and vivid versus all the parties and potato chip memories I've accumulated over the past half-century? Emotionally, it was a big deal. I achieved a new status level by being allowed to stay up late. There was excitement in the air; my parents didn't entertain that much. I was treated to a snack after dinner, a rare occasion indeed. Grownups lavished me with attention; there were no cousins to compete for hugs. I felt warm, snuggly and safe in the night. No imagined nighttime monsters would dare invade a home filled with so many noisy grownups.

Today, I triggered that memory when I treated myself to potato chips at an out-of-the-ordinary snack time, accompanied by other cues, such as snuggling up on the warm and cozy sofa, and switching on the TV. In the action of making this memory tonight, I was reinforcing the first one made long before my conscious mind was developed. In the first memory, as at this moment, logical considerations such as calories, healthiness, timing of the snack, are no match for the instant gratification and the powerful emotion of feeling loved, warm and safe after a lousy day at work in the big, bad world.

It doesn't matter whether or not we can consciously recall those initial, high impact subconscious memories. They are there in you and in the patient you are caregiving.

Because I make my living as a writer, I'm more skilled than most at knowing my cues and triggering the detailed recall of these subconscious memories. I've practiced it. But this is a skill that can be learned. It's especially important if you're caregiving someone with whom you've lived a lifetime.

It's like searching for buried treasure. Each memory is linked with many other memories, emotions and behaviors. If you'll recall, my memory starred my parents, brother, relatives and Lawrence Welk's champagne music-makers. It featured the feel of flannel PJ's with feet, the scent of bubble bath, the sight of party lights, the sound of music, as well as the taste of potato chips. It was accompanied by good behavior. I toddled off to bed and promptly fell asleep. And all of these tiny memories have their own memory trees and are linked to similar emotional memories (with or without potato chips) throughout the years.

For caregiving, I can take advantage of the unique way the subconscious mind stores long-term memories. I can switch my approach from teaching Eve the multitude of tasks she needs to function in life, to helping her remember consciously or subconsciously how she used to be. I do this by creating activities that touch past emotional memories and the associated behaviors.

If you ever saw the classic movie *The Miracle Worker* (the Helen Keller story), you'll remember the exciting climax. Deaf and blind Helen finally connected the finger language word she was learning to the real world. In a Eureka! style moment, she realized that the finger word for water meant the same thing as the cool liquid gushing out of the water pump. That triggered her subconscious memory, and she somehow remembered the only word she had spoken in her life—"wa-wa"—at age six months. It was the link that made sense of all the finger words she was being taught. At last, her conscious mind understood what her subconscious had known for years. It was waiting to be triggered by an intuitive teacher with a technique that connected the subconscious mind to the "conscious" world.

For brain caregiving, you are that teacher and your textbooks are all the memories you can find, touch or cue, and transform into Eureka! memories today. You don't even have to be consciously aware of the memories. You will do your guessing in accordance with the subconscious mind's other astounding attribute. The subconscious is also the keeper of the personal value and belief system to ensure survival of the mind, body and spirit.

In order to embark on this memory treasure hunt, we'll need to know both the caregiver's and the patient's motivations—the reason to wake up in the morning and keep on keeping on—no matter what the rest of the world deems a success. It's who we are at the core. Since our life situations have changed so drastically and dramatically with the brain trauma and our new roles as patient and caregiver, we must revisit our concept of who we are and why.

At this juncture, I think it's important for you to know how I learned all about the "mumbo-jumbo" subconscious mind many, many years ago.

As I discussed in *Brain, Heal Thyself*, I have been a student of the subconscious mind for years. I first learned about it in an adult education class that taught relaxation and creative visualization for stress control. Later my friend, Dr. Lawrence Beuret, taught me about the role of the subconscious mind in his work with psychosomatic illnesses, phobias, addictions and post-traumatic stress disorder. (I was writing informational brochures to educate his patients.)

Unfortunately, the doctor was not available when I set up my home rehabilitation program for Eve. Thankfully, I remembered what he had taught me so I could incorporate it into my caregiving strategy. (You can read Dr. Beuret's in-depth explanation of the subconscious mind in my first book.) Technical considerations aside, it is more important for you to know what my belief system was—because that is the basis for the Eureka! strategy.

Thus, I believed: The subconscious mind stores all conscious and unconscious memories from birth, including the information supplied by all five senses. The greater the emotional impact of a memory, the easier it is to consciously recall. Memories are linked by emotional association. Besides emotional content, memories contain information gleaned from the five senses and concurrent thoughts. These can be linked, too. (For example, the smell of burning leaves can trigger a memory of a school book report homework assignment, as well as the feeling of entering a cozy house on a chilly autumn day.)

The subconscious mind's operation is based on belief, and not necessarily on fact. Everything the subconscious mind does comes from its primary mission: to protect whatever that person believes is necessary for survival—spiritually and emotionally as well as physically. The subconscious mind communicates through hunches, inspirations, body language, feelings, visualizations and dreams, including daydreams. It prefers visual over written and verbal communication. It is not logical; it is emotion-based and literal.

With all of this collected wisdom on the subconscious mind, I eventually arrived at the conclusion that Eve's subconscious was trying to help her survive physically, mentally and emotionally. If I appealed to it—and communicated with it correctly—then Eve's subconscious would be persuaded to cooperate with my rehab ideas. It would help me help Eve rewire her brain. Furthermore, if I could tap into Eve's subconscious memory storage and evoke a nice, juicy memory, then perhaps I could also bring back the behavior that was taking place at the time the memory was first made.

Likewise, I might also bring back the behaviors associated with all of the memories that have linked to that initial memory throughout Eve's lifetime. This premise is the foundation of the rehabilitation aspect of the Eureka! strategy.

Don't you think this is beginning to sound more like common sense than mumbo-jumbo? Everyone has a subconscious mind, wherever or whatever it is, whether or not we put it to practical use. The problem is that our sophisticated, statistical-oriented, proof-driven system of healthcare doesn't have the time (or more importantly, money) to devote itself to this nebulous research. Let's face it—our healthcare industry focuses on pharmaceuticals and procedures that can be tested because we as patients and caregivers demand certainty, proof and seals of approval. It's not a bad thing. I'd like proof, too. Unfortunately, not much can be proven about recovering a brain, at least not in my lifetime—or Eve's. My intuition tells me that the development of emotion-based, subconscious-oriented brain rehabilitation therapies for home use is years away. Sadly, but logically, my analytical conscious mind agrees.

I believe it is the caregiver's duty to check this or any home strategy with a medical professional. Yes, I've checked out my strategy with several doctors, but as long as Eve is in good physical shape, they don't seem too interested in my little home strategies for Eve's emotional/cognitive health. Any mention of the subconscious mind merits little more than a doubtful nod and an emotional pat on the head, as in "You go, girl."

However, as you read on, you'll see how the Eureka! strategy developed and worked for Eve and me, thanks to the function, design and capabilities of the ever-elusive subconscious mind.

SUGGESTION:

In one of your quiet moments, try to conjure up a few really old (positive) favorite memories, especially those shared with the patient. Try to recall the incident. What did you taste, smell, touch, hear or see? How did you feel? Happy, sad, loved, safe, accepted, good, courageous, etc? That's it for now. Enjoy your stroll down memory lane.

8

Intuition Tells Me You're Intuitive, Too

Looking back, I can see that the problem I had communicating with Eve was what started me thinking about including the subconscious mind in my rehabilitation strategy.

For the first few years, conversing with Eve was on par with talking to the wall. Most of the time Eve's eyes were lifeless. She had to be told to look at me. When I did have her attention, I had to talk fast, before her focus floated over my head, taking her concentration with it. She had acquired a most-annoying habit of yawning as her concentration waned. It seemed as if what I was saying was terrifically boring. Actually, it was boring, as far as I was concerned; so this made the whole process that much more irritating and frustrating.

I found myself taking three deep breaths before I attempted any lengthy instructions (more than two sentences). I wanted to slow down, pace myself, get in tune with her rhythm and energy level. I had to work at this. Perhaps other caregivers do it more naturally. For me, this was the first step to aligning my subconscious mind with Eve's. As we will see, that enabled me to create the environment where I could intuitively communicate with her.

While I was concentrating on my breathing and slowing myself down to Eve's speed, I was simultaneously increasing my awareness of Eve's eyes, face, body and the energy (or lack thereof) that she was giving off. Though her attention span was still very short, I was better able to gauge her level of comprehension and her interest in what I was saying. I could tell when I could push her and when I couldn't. Though her unchanging facial expression was generally sweet, almost smiling, I could pick up on the slightest tics and grimaces of irritation, furrowing of a brow in worry, knitting of eyebrows for a question, darting of eyes that signified bathroom time. The big bonus was that now I could also pick up on that glint in her eyes, that spark, that light, that told me she understood what I was saying and she was ready to learn more.

One day I received a phone call from a faraway friend of Eve's, who was also a veteran caregiver of her brain-damaged son, a car crash survivor. I was grateful for her ongoing support. I was also a little bit envious that in her household there were two people (she and her husband) sharing the caregiving duties. Anyway, as the phone conversation was winding down, I said, "I have to check Eve's diaper."

Eve's friend said, "I thought she was wearing protective underpants."

"Well, yeah, if that's what you want to call those big fluffy things. I call 'em diapers with leg holes," I replied.

"You should treat Eve with more respect," her friend admonished. "They're protective underpants. That's what you should tell Eve."

This was a semantic challenge that would normally spur the old me into verbal fisticuffs. Amazingly, I retreated with a vague response and said, "It was great of you to call."

When I hung up from the mostly very supportive phone call, I realized how very sensitive I was to her caregiving criticism. She made me angry. I wondered why. Though I normally don't like criticism, I usually accept it with the attitude of "Take what you need and leave the rest." But fifteen minutes after the call, I was still bristling and arguing with her in my head.

After further thought I came to the conclusion that I couldn't afford to pay attention to anyone who criticized the way I talked with uncommunicative Eve. Obviously, at some point I had sub-consciously decided to communicate on an intuitive level with Eve. This meant that I should absolutely not change my style of con-versing—my choice of words or my way of expressing whatever I wanted to say. I intuitively knew that if Eve was okay, she would agree with me that the protective underwear was a glorified dia-per and that putting on the darned things was a "pain in the butt." (Pun intended.)

So I made an important pact with myself that day to maintain the "old" way of conversing with Eve, thereby freeing me from having to change my style. I did give my subconscious a message to watch what I said to her in public. But I truly, truly believed that maintaining my "old" style of communicating—meaning the rhythm, tone and selection of my words—was imperative for bring-ing back the "old" talkative, always-joking Eve. If Eve had selected the "old" me as her friend many years ago, she certainly wouldn't want to wake up to find that I had turned into one of those mushy, compliant, sweet-talking caregivers today.

For most of the first eighteen months, even when directly ques-tioned, Eve was unable to tell me if she was hot, cold, uncomfort-able, sleepy, or that she felt an urge "to go." As time progressed, I could answer these questions just by looking at her. Meanwhile, I was also learning how to put myself in the relaxed, intuitive state, no matter what task I was doing. In other words, I started picking up on her energy shift, even in another room.

As time went on, I gained confidence in the process. I could relax even more. I was learning to trust my intuition. This ability spread to all sorts of situations; but by far its most important appli-cation was in communicating with Eve.

We all have intuition; it comes with being human. Surely at some point you've said, "I had a feeling this would be a great day" or "I know I can find a parking space closer to the door." By defin-ition, intuition is simply the immediate perceiving, or knowing something, without using the (logical) conscious mind.

Lest you get the wrong impression, I didn't spend the days waltzing around the house in a "woo-woo" state, nodding to flickering candles on my left and an incense burner on the right, checking to see if Buddha Eve was glowing. I'm far too practical for that.

But I knew that my purposeful daily relaxation routine (which I had been faithfully practicing) was beginning to pay off. With my calmer emotions and stress-control program in effect, I could feel my awareness level rise, my sensitivity to slight changes increase. The more I trusted my intuition, the stronger it became.

We're speaking relatively here. In "regular" life, I am always thinking. It's an exhausting habit. I'd be willing to bet that half the caregiver population is naturally more relaxed than I am. Those who are more relaxed naturally have a big head start on me for using intuition as a tool for caregiving and rehabilitation.

Prior to perfecting my intuitive communication skills, I had been using intuition in spurts throughout Eve's hospitalization. After all, Eve had been in a comatose state for two months, followed by another month of the inability to talk due to her paralyzed vocal chords.

Initially, intuition became part of my caregiving/rehabilitation routine when Eve was still in a coma in the nursing home. Back then I intuitively decided to try rousing her from the coma only when I sensed a rise in her energy, usually accompanied by a shift in her sleeping position or a sleepy little cough. With practice, I became an expert at guessing when my attempts to rouse her had a good chance at succeeding. Then I'd be rewarded by her open eyes and a fleeting feeling that she recognized me for fifteen seconds or so before she lapsed back into her subconscious dreamland.

Later, I relied on intuition to communicate with her in the home caregiving situation. I invoked that sixth sense to guess (often correctly) when Eve was cold, hot, needed the bathroom or wanted to eat. Many months later, I used intuition to guess which Eureka! activities would work best for Eve in any given situation.

Way back in my younger days, I never, ever thought I had the "power of intuition." I thought it was a talent or skill reserved for gifted psychics. I wasn't too sure I wanted to have intuition—let alone devote my time to developing it.

It was my creative visualization teacher, the one who taught the course on using relaxation for stress control, who changed my mind. She offered an advanced class to study the relationship between intuition and relaxation. Initially, I told her I had better things to do with my time; but she convinced me it might be fun to explore the remote possibility I had intuition.

She was planning to host the advanced class in her home. Truthfully, that made me curious. I wondered if she had crystal chandeliers in every room. I also recall the price was right, seven bucks a session. Little did I know it was one of the best investments I ever made in my life.

During these classes, mostly composed of regular people like me who didn't think they had an intuitive bone in their bodies, we explored some interesting topics. One evening session was devoted to attempting to "read" the energy levels emitted by each person, also known as auras. I had no idea if I was "reading" my class-mates correctly, but we all had fun pretending and guessing. What was weird was that, more often than not, the majority of us agreed that so-and-so had more or less energy than the other so-and-so we were "reading."

Was this simply coincidence? Perhaps. However, the ability to read variable, personal, energy levels sure came in handy when I was attempting to rouse Eve from her coma.

One night we played a different game in the advanced class. Most of us in the class were strangers to each other. For this game, the teacher took advantage of that fact. She paired up two strangers and told the pair to find a place to sit together somewhere in the room. I was paired with a woman in her thirties. I knew her first name, but that was all. At first glance I noted she was attractive, well-dressed, and had a nice hairdo. She looked intelligent and seemed quite friendly. (Little did I know that, even at this point, some of those observations were intuitive.)

As the teacher instructed, we sat on a couch, facing each other. For the first minute, we were told to quietly stare into our partner's eyes. This made everyone a little self-conscious. You could hear sporadic nervous giggles around the room.

The teacher made us get our acts together. "Relax," she commanded. "Take three breaths and be quiet." She paused and continued. "Now I want you to imagine taking your new friend on a little day trip. You can go anywhere in the world. Or you can rocket to the moon if you want. You can stay in the present or time travel to the past or future. The only rule is that you imagine as many details as you can: where you are, what you see, hear, taste, touch. Most importantly, I want you to imagine how you feel on the outing."

Ever-negative, my first thought was that this exercise wasn't going to work. Oh, what the heck, I might as well play along.

And so I imagined that my new friend and I met in the local suburban Chicago train depot and boarded the train for downtown Chicago. When we reached our destination, we walked the long walk to Michigan Avenue, Chicago's magnificent mile. Once there, we strolled over the river bridge to one of my favorite restaurants, Jacques. At that time, it had one of the few outdoor dining setups in the area, a garden dining atrium. After dining on a fresh luncheon salad, we walked across the Avenue. We entered Water Tower Place, with all of its upscale shops. For the rest of the afternoon, we window-shopped, tried on hats, clothes, shoes and then we called it a day.

The teacher called out, "Time's up," jolting me and my partner out of our day dream revelry. The teacher announced, "Now I want each of you to report on your outing. Madonna, we'll begin with you."

Why pick on me, I wondered. I sighed and proceeded to dutifully report on my excursion to the class. When I reached the end I editorialized a little. "What's really dumb and weird about this adventure was that I had a lot of fun. Normally, I would never take the train into Chicago; I prefer driving. I wouldn't order a healthy salad; I'd order meat for lunch. Though I do enjoy visiting Water Tower Place, I wouldn't plan a day of shopping. I'd rather go to the Art Institute and look at Impressionist paintings. So I don't think I did this adventure correctly because . . . ."

I stopped talking because I happened to glance at my partner at that moment. She was sitting there wide-eyed and open-mouthed. She looked as though she had just seen a ghost. I had to laugh. "Your turn," I gamefully tossed the ball to my partner.

And so she described her adventure. "It was a sunny morning. Madonna came to my house in Arlington Heights, just down the road from the train station. We drove downtown in my car. Odd, because I don't like to drive. Our first stop was Water Tower Place, where we went to a restaurant for lunch. It was that glorified deli sandwich place, D. B. Kaplan. Need I say that I would have preferred a luscious salad at Jacques. Afterward, we window-shopped the exclusive stores, which was my favorite part of the day. But we couldn't stay long because we had to walk down Michigan Avenue to visit the Art Institute. We wanted to see the Renoir exhibit before it closed."

Boo! It was my turn to see the ghost. I couldn't believe it. Not only was there a shocking similarity in our imaginary adventures, but every single pair of strangers in the class—seven of them—had similar accounts. One pair went for a balloon ride together, another visited the moon, and one pair traveled back in time to sit around the campfire inside their Stone Age cave.

Oh, it was eerie. I have never forgotten that night. In fact, I remembered it again one morning when I was staring into the vacant eyes of Eve, wondering if there was anything left inside her broken brain. And even if there was something there, how in the world would I be able to reach it?

Yes, at first glance, developing intuition seems to be a useless parlor game. If I hadn't depended on intuition as a tool in those early recovery days, I doubt I would have had a book to write. Speaking purely from intuition, I doubt there would be much to report about Eve's recovery.

Developing intuition actually requires very little purposeful time investment. I started developing mine by guessing what was in the mailbox, who was calling on the phone (before caller I.D. was invented), whether a certain friend would call, if I could find a close parking space, and what the weather would be. (That's more of a challenge in the Midwest than in most areas of the country.) Then I would make a mental note of right versus wrong guesses.

That's it. I've played the intuition game all of my life; but never were the stakes as high as my need to use my intuition for caregiving.

SUGGESTION:

I suggest you try developing your intuition by guessing—not trying to control—what might happen during the day. Guess what the weather will be. Guess what's in the mailbox. Who cares if you're right or wrong? You're just practicing.

Next, try guessing what people are thinking. Observe their body language. Try to feel the energy of the situation. Hopefully, some of those situations will allow you to ask the other person whether or not your guess is right.

If it is, stick a feather in your cap. If not, well, try, try again. Someday very soon you'll realize how very intuitive you've become.

9

Do I Really Want to Be a Caregiver?

It was New Year's Eve, 2002. Eve and I weren't going out anywhere. Our days of boisterous celebration were long past. Nevertheless, I tried to get in the spirit of the holiday by dedicating a page in my journal/notebook to New Year's resolutions. But the words that flowed from my pen sounded more like a question to the universe. "Why am I a caregiver? This is not the reason I moved to Door County. I wanted to be an artist. What's to become of me?"

Then came a flood of questions and lame excuses posing as answers. "Why don't you paint? I'm not inspired. Then why don't you get a job? There are none in this tourist area during the winter. Everyone's in Florida anyway. (All rise to observe a minute of pity for the winter-weary caregiver.) So why don't you move back to Chicago and get a big job? I can't; that's why I moved out of Chicago. So why not get a little job? And do what with Eve? Hiring a sitter will cost more than I'll make. You know, you're getting fat. Go on a diet. Why don't you shut up? Face it; you don't know what you want to do."

That last statement was painfully true, I admitted to myself as I grabbed a leftover Christmas cookie. I've been so goal-oriented all my life that day-to-day living without pursuing a carrot seemed meaningless. I would not allow myself the goal of rehabilitating Eve. I had no reason to believe that Eve was going to get any better. No medical person had given me hope that anything I could do would make any difference. And I certainly had no credentials or experience to logically challenge that.

I knew I couldn't leave Eve alone. I doubted she could make it a week on her own (and that was being generous). On the other hand, patient care, physical therapy, domestic service were way at the bottom of my career choice list. If I was going to stay with Eve, I had to find my motivation for getting up each day.

As I munched more cookies, I returned to memories of my college days. Way back then, I took enough psychology courses to earn a minor in it. But did I remember anything from them? Not really. What I recalled was that the courses and schoolbooks were filled with dozens of experiments, statistical results and—to my mind—predictable conclusions based on common sense. (Of course a rat will learn how to navigate his way through a maze if a piece of cheese is waiting at the end. I would, too.)

I was very disappointed that the study of human psychology was limited, at the undergraduate level, to memorizing mostly common sense theories with little practical application in my life. However, one psychological theory, Maslow's Theory of Human Motivations, came alive when it was presented in my advertising communications class. Now here was a theory that had meaning in real life. Leave it to the advertising people to put a "spin" on a psychological theory and use it as "proof" that their creative approaches to selling cars, cake mixes and toilet paper have scientific validity.

In that spirit, allow me to summarize Maslow's theory (the way I remembered it) and show how I applied it to advertising, and later to my New Year's resolutions and my caregiving situation.

Here goes. Human needs can be divided into five levels. A pyramid is often used to demonstrate this. The bottom level represents physical needs: food, shelter, and clothing. The next level is safety: financial security, good health, etc. These needs have to be satisfied in order to proceed up the pyramid. This is followed by the satisfaction of social needs: peer acceptance, marriage and family, sexual and nonsexual love. The next level is self-esteem: self-respect through achievement in one's profession and one's role in society. The ultimate motivation is self-actualization: realizing one's potential. In theory, this need is only addressed after all the lower-level needs are satisfied.

Actually, there are several psychologists who disagree that there is a hierarchy of human needs. But for my purposes as a career ad writer—and now as a caregiver—the theory is a very helpful tool. It forces me to be aware and considerate of people's motivations, including my own and Eve's.

My point to caregivers is this: If we are going to do this job, this new mission in life, it's important to know why we're doing it. If you are caring for the love of your life and you have no more dreams to be fulfilled, go for it. For the rest of us, who don't find total fulfillment in caregiving, read on.

We all need a reason to wake up in the morning. Let's presume you are already doing the best you can to provide food, shelter, clothing, safety and financial security. You know your situation. If that pursuit isn't taking all your time or attention, then you need to determine your higher motivations—wishes, dreams, goals—to give the day meaning.

How do you do this? Take a "time out." Now, realize what it is that has motivated you throughout your life at your highest, most interesting, most exciting level of motivation. Even if it's a dream you've only been working toward—list it.

Now the question for me was: can any of my lifetime goals be achieved while I am caregiving Eve? If yes, then can this caregiving situation help me achieve my goals, perhaps in a unique way?

Before I explain how this line of questioning relates to caregiver motivation, let's look at how it plays in the creation of an advertising commercial.

Back in the early 1970s, if an advertiser wanted to sell a luxury American car, the TV commercial looked like this: A silver-haired man in a three-piece business suit drives his luxury car up to the entrance of a posh hotel and tosses his keys to the awestruck valet. Then he rounds the car to open the door for his impossibly chic young wife (read girlfriend), while a foursome of vacationing guys pause enroute to the golf course to admire his girlfriend/car. Back then, such a commercial would capture the attention and appeal to the self-actualization needs of most of the potential luxury car buyers. In 60 seconds it told the audience that this man had already satisfied his needs of food, shelter and clothing. He had financial security, success in career, provided for wife and family, earned respect and had self-esteem. Now he had just driven up to the hotel in his statement of self-actualization. What better way to prove that one has arrived than to buy a status symbol, such as a luxury car?

In the 21st century, this is still a valid creative motivational approach, except that the commercial does little to motivate entire groups of potential buyers—women, for example. Their needs and their motivations are different. In fact, such an ignorant commercial could potentially alienate women and persons of color, by insinuating that success was only reserved for middle-aged, white males. I'd be willing to bet that years of seeing such commercials actually drive successful women to buy a "foreign" car instead of the American brand that was burdened with so many appeals aimed at traditional white male needs.

Now what does all this have to do with caregiving? Well, let's just examine my skewed picture of what a real caregiver should be. Having watched a lifetime of movie and TV scenarios featuring the typical caregiver, I believe a stereotype (mainly from the 1950s, '60s and '70s) was created in my mind.

This movie star stereotype is sweet, kind, loving and very patient. No doubt, the afflicted one is her spouse. The caregiver is old and comfortably situated. She isn't fretting about food, shelter, clothing, personal safety or financial security. Her lifetime goal— raising the children—has been achieved. At this very moment, those children are waiting in the wings to provide support, along with a slew of neighbors and friends holding casseroles and cakes.

Meanwhile, the patient is appreciative and motivated to get well, even if the cards are stacked against him. There's little discussion of the patient's behavior being unmanageable. With the help and support of loved ones, the viewer has no doubt that the heroine can hang on a few months, until the end.

How could a stroke/brain trauma caregiver (like me) relate to this? How could this motivate me?

Most all stroke/brain trauma caregivers are not dealing with patients who are deteriorating. The patient's mind and body have already survived the worst of the devastation, physically, mentally, emotionally.

On one hand, this situation is good because obviously there's hope for recovery. But the not so good news is that modern medicine isn't sure how to rehabilitate most physical, mental, emotional disabilities. Paralysis? Aphasia? Memory restoration? Nobody knows for sure how to bring anything back.

The situation gives the home caregiver a false sense of hope and power. Yes, the things a caregiver does can possibly contribute to the patient's recovery. But no one knows for sure what the caregiver should do, or if the caregiver is capable. No one with credentials will promise any sort of good outcome. Consequently, the caregiver is overwhelmed by many rehabilitation choices and little professional direction on how to devote time and effort. Which disability does the caregiver fix first—the chicken or the egg?

That's the situation in which I found myself. The only control I had was over my decisions and actions. I still wasn't very motivated to be a classic caregiver, yet I wouldn't abandon my friend. I knew I would have to guard against entertaining unreasonable expectations or hope for my friend's recovery, or else face my personal consequences of frustration, stress and, inevitably, debilitating depression.

Meanwhile, I still needed a reason (a motivation) to get up tomorrow and the next day. I still had lots of needs, desires and wishes that had nothing to do with the caregiving situation. What I had to concentrate on and reinforce were the motivations that could help me become the person I always wanted to be, and simultaneously continue to serve as a caregiver or, as I was beginning to realize, a brain rehabilitator.

I chose these two longtime needs (motivations) to implement for my daily inspiration: First, for as long as I could remember, the need to communicate—to express myself through art and writing—has dominated my life. I believe the communication process involves teaching and learning in equal measure. For me, the teaching aspect involves creativity. I thrive on that never-ending search for the logical words, emotional appeals and visual triggers that attract attention and make the message memorable. As for the learning aspect, I believe listening is the key. Developing intuition and practicing relaxation would help me improve my listening ability. No doubt about it; learning how to harness intuition for brain healing was a fascinating challenge. Yes, this will become my motivation for my role in Eve's rehabilitation routine.

My other motivation is grounded in my desire to live a sober and serene life and to give back to those who made my recovered life worth living. To my thinking, I can say "thank you" until I'm blue in the face. For me, the only way to express gratitude is to give something of myself to someone in need. So my motivation here is to give back primarily to Eve, in a way that does not undermine my serenity (freedom from frustration, stress of expectations, and depression) or threaten my sobriety. I trust I will know my limits and protect myself. It would be great if this way of life could also help me achieve the ultimate goal—one day at a time.

So now I have my personal motivations. Surprisingly, as I write my motivations in my journal, it looks like the recipe for Maslow's highest level of need/motivation: self-actualization. I mean, it appears I'm describing the person I always wanted to be.

Wow! Thanks, Eve. I guess I really am motivated to be a brain rehabilitator.

SUGGESTION:

Now is a good time to take a look at your lifetime goals and motivations.

If you know your goals, that's great. Write them down, let them rest overnight and look at them again in the morning light to see if there's anything you would change.

If you've never done an exercise such as this, here's how to get started. List these categories: physical health, relationships, profession, finances, hobbies/recreation, spiritual. Write a single sentence describing where you would like to be growth-wise in each category by this time next year.

Look for those goals that you share with the patient or relate to your caregiving role in any way. Highlight those goals, just for your information.

Next, share your findings with a caring friend or counselor. (Announcing your intention to another human being often helps reinforce your motivation to achieve a goal.)

Review your goals often until you have a clear picture of what you want your life to be in a year. Always keep in mind that you really can't control your patient's rate of recovery. However, you can control your thoughts, actions and emotional reactions to the happenings in your life.

10

To Be or Not to Be a Lonely Caregiver

No doubt about it, caregiving is much easier to do using a team approach. But what if one doesn't have family or close friends who are willing or able to participate in the process?

I can empathize. Eve and I had isolated ourselves in a rural community, five hours away from our lifelong home in Chicago. During our first year in our new home, Eve and I hadn't made any close friends. I wasn't in a position to start making friends now. Fortunately, the few local people we had met were generous and charitable beyond the call of neighborliness. But I needed even more help and it was up to me to establish my own support network. There are no rewards for the lonely caregiver who insists on handling the situation all by herself.

Oh, sure, there was enough activity to keep me going through Eve's early days of recovery. I was busy visiting Eve in the nursing home and hospitals, accompanying her to professional rehab, checking out all the social services she wasn't eligible to receive, and dealing with bill collectors who called me daily for a "chat." But it didn't take me long to discover that late at night, an hour or so after I put Eve to bed, loneliness would hit me like a sledge-hammer. And then, it was too late to call anyone in Chicago for help. Long distance phone service may have been cheaper at night way back then, but I couldn't think of too many friends who wanted to be awakened by my midnight whining.

It was up to me to put together my own support network—first, to survive emotionally, and secondarily, to fire up my enthusiasm.

Yes, I would have preferred to keep my problems in the family; but I had to look elsewhere. I was blessed with several friends who had successfully survived life's challenges. I was also grateful that they were willing to share their experience, strength and hope. For instance, one of Eve's closest friends in Chicago made it her mission to keep me going. She installed an outgoing 800 number so she could call me twice a day to deliver a pep talk. I swear her calls kept me sane, sober and serene on those long, dark nights when it seemed nothing I could do with Eve would make a difference. But at other times, I had to ask for help.

Asking for help becomes easier when you consider how quickly loneliness can easily lead to self-destructive bad habits. I'll do anything to thwart this progression and to nip this situation in the bud, even if it means phone calls or emails to people I barely know just to gain an ounce of support. Why? Because once I start finding relief in bad habits, it rapidly leads to addiction (a state where a bad habit takes on a life of its own).

Not everyone is "blessed" with an addictive tendency; but its cousins—depression, despair and obsessive/compulsive behavior— are no trip to Hollywood either. All of them rob the caregiver of that precious energy and enthusiasm for everyday living.

Isolated and unapproachable, a caregiver stands little chance of receiving outside intervention to end the bad habits or addictions. After all, who's going to confront the caregiver on an addiction when there's a chance they might have to assume the caregiving duties while the caregiver gets some professional help? The caregiver begins to welcome the isolation as the bad habit or addiction demands more and more time. Meanwhile, the patient's not getting better and now the caregiver's sick, too.

What are these bad habits that lurk in the shadows, waiting to pounce on an unsuspecting caregiver? Overeating, under eating, nonstop TV watching and computer gaming or Internet surfing; not to mention casino/Internet gambling, alcoholism and prescription drug abuse (anti-anxiety meds and sleeping aids). Though maybe not exactly addictive, obsessive thinking (worrying too much) isn't any fun, either.

It's worth the effort to stop the situation before it ever begins. In fact, it hardly takes any effort at all if one is willing to be honest with a couple of friends. Choosing the friends you'll confide in requires thoughtful consideration. They may or may not be your impulsive first choice. In other words, your best golfing buddy, favorite neighbor, or adult child may not be good choices. A caregiver cannot ask for this sort of help from those who will pity, or play power games, or who have similar unchecked problems.

For example, your three hundred pound aunt is not the best source for support if you fear you're on the verge of any type of eating disorder. Nor is your happy-go-lucky, card-playing buddy the best one to consult if you fear your frequent trips to a local casino might soon become a gambling problem. And let's keep in mind that obsessively searching the Internet for answers to all our problems can lead to addiction, too.

Take it from me, addiction can be very sneaky. It doesn't care how nice or good or well-meaning you are—or want to be. Remember when I mentioned how stress caused me to start grinding my teeth right after I had suffered a debilitating bout with a bad back? Well, I didn't tell you that the dentist recommended the highly addictive painkiller, Vicodin, to deal with the agonizing pain the teeth-grinding caused. Usually, I'll refuse it, because of the very real possibility it can lead me back into mood-altering addictions. But I couldn't stand the pain. (I had aggravated my teeth nerves and it felt like three toothaches at once.) I told the dentist okay, but limit my prescription to three days worth. Then I went home and dutifully called my 12-Step sponsor and a local friend and told them what I was taking and for how long. Honesty isn't fun for me; it's simply a survival tool.

For people with any inclination to addictive or obsessive behavior, it's best to call someone who is wise to the ways of addiction or obsession. Then ask if they'll be your new best friend for a while. Add that person to your support network, along with those friends/acquaintances who've overcome life's tragedies. You can ask them to tell their stories again, but this time take notes. No caregiver task is as important as establishing a support network of friends, family and acquaintances.

The good news is that once the problem of caregiver isolation is recognized and action is taken to correct the situation, that process automatically inspires an attitude of gratitude for help from friends. That in turn generates enthusiasm for meeting the challenges life has presented.

If we're trying to inspire a loved one with a disabled brain to meet his or her greatest challenge, the least we can do is try to serve as an example of what inspired living might offer. We expect our loved one to ask for help when needed; we should be willing to do the same.

Now is the time to get in shape. Soon we'll be assuming the role as the Pied Piper of the Eureka! strategy and we'll need lots of enthusiasm to do it.

SUGGESTION:

If you have close family or friends, ask for help. If you don't, join an online support system, such as my website, Eurekamaster.com. Here's another idea. Find somebody that both of you, caregiver and patient, can help. Volunteer an hour a week to give back to someone else. Certainly your local hospital, YMCA, church or humane society, would welcome your help. If you haven't started it, try my gratitude-with-a-twist list for a week.

11

What Motivates the Patient?

Now it's time to figure out the patient's motivations. It doesn't matter how well the patient is functioning; I believe it's a worthwhile exercise. It's easier to teach—to inspire—re-learning when the rewards are framed in the context of motivations that the patient has always held dear.

Admittedly, neither Eve nor I were motivated by the same things that traditionally motivate many women our age. Many women believe that mothering and raising children (including grandchildren) and providing a home for a husband and family are the major motivations of their lives. Providing for a family and achieving success in a career are mega-motivators for more men than women. If any of these fit your patient, you're halfway to discovering the motivational basis for your Eureka! strategy. This is not a study in psychology. It's plain old-fashioned common sense.

In our case, I do not believe Eve comprehended the concept of motivation in the early years of brain recovery. However, that did not stop me from discussing it with her regularly. If I paid attention during these mostly one-way conversations, I could pick up subtle cues and clues (facial expressions, body language, shifts in energy) that could tell me if I was on the right track. Yes, I was relying on intuition; but it was surprising how much input Eve gave me.

(Apparently the aneurysm never affected her ability to roll her eyes at me if she disagreed.)

Right off the bat, I could anticipate problems in applying Maslow's hierarchy of needs for motivating Eve. Certainly, the primary needs of food, shelter, clothing and personal safety were being provided by me. So Eve didn't "need" them. However, in the event of my untimely demise, I doubted she would be motivated to provide them for herself—even if the solutions to her problems were as close as the refrigerator or hanging in the closet.

Actually, I have a sneaking suspicion that a "tough love" attitude might be the best motivator. In other words, I should leave her alone for a couple of days to see if she could fend for herself. I'm not that tough yet. However, if I could find someone to watch her at a distance, I might try that. For now, I will not risk Eve's health or safety in order to teach her how to cope with a situation that doesn't exist. I have to trust my intuition that I'm doing the right thing right now. We have plenty of current needs to challenge Eve's brain.

So, let's return to Maslow's hierarchy. Maslow noted that once those basic needs were fulfilled and a person was operating on a higher motivation level, that person would continue to function at that level, even if satisfying those physiological needs suddenly became a priority. For example, theoretically a businessman whose house was foreclosed would find a way to show up at work—showered, shaved and suited—even though he was homeless. An artist would subsist on beans in order to afford the art supplies he required to continue painting.

This is the quirk in the theory that I had to apply to Eve's rehabilitation strategy. Eve apparently did not perceive any threat or change to her basic physiological status. Therefore, I believed she was still operating at a higher level of motivation that had propelled her through the years preceding the aneurysm.

The challenge was to select those motivations. For that, I relied on remembering the stories she had told me before the aneurysm—

her accounts of the most significant, meaningful and emotional events of her life.

In reality, I was just guessing. But that didn't matter because, if I was wrong, it would become apparent soon enough. Eve simply wouldn't be motivated and I'd have to go through my guessing process again.

Happily, it appeared the motivations I selected were more right than wrong. I determined that Eve's four major motivating factors in her life were: her desire to participate in theater productions; her desire to perpetuate the experience of her college year in Rome, Italy, by continuing to explore the arts and everything European; her desire to create a happy home for family; and her desire to make a good marriage. I selected the first three as the platform to stage her recovery. Since her husband was deceased, I didn't want to chance stumbling upon painful memories.

I also tried one other motivator that would have worked splendidly with me had our roles been reversed. Since Eve and her mom had shared a house (until Mom's death) and had taken many trips together, including excursions to New York for Broadway theater productions, I "assumed" that Eve would want to please her mom. (After all, I still wanted to please my mother and she had been gone 20 years.)

It wasn't that Eve didn't love her mom; but I now understand that their relationship had been quite passive-aggressive. I didn't learn this until the tenth time I petitioned Eve to make her bed the way her mom taught her, or to dress up nicely as she would for a visit from Mom. It took a while, but I finally got the message that dear, sweet Mom was definitely out as a motivator for Eve.

Considering our dire financial situation post-aneurysm, money should also be a major motivator for Eve. Though I continue to regularly inform Eve of her financial situation, it never seems to bother her. If I felt she comprehended it gut-level, I believe I could use it to motivate behavior changes or learning. Interestingly, she does sense her dire predicament, in the event something happens to me.

She remembers what to do "in case of." She also comprehends helping me earn an income. If I ask for help typing or editing a free-lance writing project, she acts motivated: She'll actually push herself when she's tired in order to help me out. But she doesn't ever seem to "believe" that her own financial situation is the same as mine (or worse).

Oh, how I wish I could use making money as a motivator for Eve. Apparently, she remembers that helping me financially was necessary to start our art gallery, the primary motivation for our move to Door County. As I described in *Brain, Heal Thyself*, Eve helped me turn our house into an art gallery—with an eye to using the home/business combo possibilities as a feature to help sell the house.

Obviously the team spirit approach worked that time. Perhaps we can do it again—and again.

SUGGESTION:

List motivations for the patient. This is the foundation for what will become your own unique Eureka! strategies for your patient.

Remember, it isn't critical to get it right the first time. You will know if you aren't motivating the patient all too soon.

Here's a little trick I borrowed from the way I plan my approach to my professional writing assignments. At night, think about the patient's motivations. List five to ten. Before you go to sleep, give yourself the suggestion that in the morning you will intuitively know which three patient motivations you can use. (If not, then just guess—and move on.)

Once you have selected the patient's motivations, trust that you will operate intuitively from this foundation with the patient's best interest at heart.

12

We Will Get Better Together

As I entered year three with Eve, it became apparent to me that "I-me-myself" was having a positive effect on Eve's recovery. No, I cannot back up my theory with scientific studies or observations. But I could see Eve's coordination, memory, cognitive and social skills were improving—not steadily, but in tiny leaps (often one step backward, two steps forward). As far as I could see, I was the major variable in the process.

In my younger days, I might have been tempted to pound my chest, Tarzan-style, and nominate myself for caregiver of the year. Instead, I was more often on my knees in humble gratitude to the 12-Step program for having taught me the mother of all motivation strategies: "We will get better together."

Here's how it works in the 12-Step program. One recovering person who has experienced success in eliminating a problem or an addiction from her life teaches a beginner how she did it. In the process, the teacher suggests a course of action she took to overcome a problem similar to the beginner's problem. The teacher doesn't offer any advice beyond her realm of personal experience. She doesn't command; she suggests a course of action for the beginner. The teacher does not take responsibility for the outcome—good or bad. It's up to the beginner to take the suggested action—or not. In the process, the beginner intuitively knows the teacher is not on a power trip and has no stake in the beginner's success or failure.

The rewards are built into the process. In the 12-Step program, both teacher and beginner benefit. The beginner learns how to live life again—minus the problem or addiction—and the teacher learns from the beginner's experience.

How does this apply to brain caregiving? No matter what problem Eve and I were tackling—physical, cognitive, emotional—I searched my background for a similar problem/experience and talked to her based on that experience. No, I had never been paralyzed (or weakened); but I had been physically challenged in my recovery from a long-ago appendectomy and a broken foot. I never was seriously cognitively impaired; but I've always been mechanically/technically dysfunctional. Handling my over-abundant emotions has been my lifelong challenge.

I can easily recall the times when I've been confused (emotionally or cognitively); I couldn't remember an event (short or long term memory loss); I've stuttered while trying to express myself; I've confabulated to fill in parts of a story to make it sound good; and I've been too anxious or exhausted to think correctly.

Relative to caregiving, I am also focusing on these 12-Step program concepts: powerlessness, acceptance, asking for help, taking action without expecting a certain result.

Here's how it plays out in our lives. Eve and I are both accepting life on life's terms and acknowledging that the patient's disabilities have adversely affected and/or challenged the patient and caregiver in different ways. Since we are not educated or trained to deal with many of the problems, we are relying on common sense, intuition, and any help the medical/social services community, family, friends or God can give us. Since we are willing to ask for help from experts, friends and God, and we know we have both the patient's and the caregiver's best interest at heart—we trust we will do the next right thing one day at a time. And last, but certainly not least, all of my past physical/mental/emotional problems, and the efforts I've made to overcome them, now become the basis for everything I am teaching Eve.

If I am actively recalling these experiences while trying to rehabilitate Eve, I will automatically be more in tune with how she views the day's challenges. Since my brain is ostensibly okay, I will hopefully be blessed with a problem-solving strategy that can work for Eve, while it makes sense for functioning in real life. In fact, I guarantee me that whatever strategy I come up with at my "buddy" level will work better than the best "advice" I could give in my role as "Queen Caregiver," as this little anecdote demonstrates.

THE BALONEY SANDWICH STORY

Making lunch was one of the first rehabilitation tasks I tried to teach Eve. I was confident that Eve could succeed because she had done it before. The occupational therapist had directed Eve to make lunch for me on the day of her graduation from outpatient rehab. As the OT explained to me, she had taught Eve to make a shopping list of ingredients for lunch. She took Eve to a store to buy them; Eve made the sandwiches, garnished them, set the table and served the luncheon to us—complete with coffee, tea and dessert.

Note: I did not actually witness the preparation process; but judging from Eve's big smile and the beaming face of the OT, I assumed that everything in the kitchen went along splendidly. This may have been my mistake.

Now grandfather's clock was chiming noon as I led Eve by the hand to our kitchen. I wasn't really hungry; yet I wanted to do everything by the book. For some reason, I was feeling nervous.

I opened the refrigerator door for Eve and, in my queenly caregiver voice commanded, "Lunch." Eve stared at the contents of the open refrigerator, and then turned to look at me. It was as if she had never before seen a refrigerator—or me. Her face was as blank as the bowl of lard on the bottom shelf. (What am I supposed to do with lard, anyway?)

I was getting cold standing there, so I grabbed the baloney, bread and mustard, and kicked the refrigerator door shut. "Here you go, Eve. Make a sandwich." Once again, she looked at me blankly. My patience was replaced by frustration.

"Pay attention," I, the Queenly Caregiver, commanded her royal subject, Eve. "Here's how to make a sandwich." I laid two slices of bread on two plates, slapped slices of baloney on top of the two, and spread mustard over the other two. "See, wasn't that easy?" I said to Eve, who was standing there like a totem pole. I took that as a yes. "So, make a cup of tea for yourself in the microwave and we'll eat lunch." The tea she could do.

We sat down at the table to eat. When we finished, I said, "So now do you remember how to do the sandwich? You did it in rehab; it's even easier at home."

She nodded and yawned, so I put her to bed for her nap. The quiet of the afternoon descended on the house, interrupted only by the more intense, dead-quiet moments (minutes?) between Eve's snores. Sleep apnea. I had no idea what to do about that, either; so I just half-heartedly listened for the next snore. Either Eve would take another breath, or she wouldn't.

However, it must've made me a little nervous because all of a sudden I had a craving for one of those little chocolate pudding cups I had bought for Eve's desserts and rewards. I headed right for the refrigerator, second shelf. They weren't there. Eve couldn't have eaten them all, could she? I looked behind the pickles and milk. Not there. I checked the other shelves. Okay, the pudding's gone. Maybe I'll have that apple I just saw. Where was it? I started looking all over again. Finally I found it.

I took it into the dining room, collapsing into the chair with a sigh. I was mildly exhausted and still aggravated about the pudding. While I munched away, it hit me. That's what the inside of that refrigerator looks like to Eve—every time she opens the door. Due to her short- or long-term memory loss, inability to perceive, focus, pay attention, recognize once-familiar objects—or due to generalized anxiety over the situation, Eve can't identify what she's looking for or remember where it is. Perhaps she can't even perceive that she's found it when she does.

Horrors! I just set up Eve for failure at lunch-making. Maybe the task is easy to relearn, but not if I confuse her while she's trying to do it.

When Eve awoke from her nap, I took her to the kitchen and sat her in front of the open refrigerator. All the items were out on the table (except for our precious ice cream). Slowly, I put everything back in the fridge, in a logical fashion that I explained to Eve every step of the way. I frequently asked her advice, whether I needed it or not. That way I could judge what's apt to confuse her in the future. By the time we were done, I had a refrigerator layout similar to the initial one; but Eve just graduated from refrigerator design 101. She had put herself on the right track for future forays into the fridge.

No, she didn't have it memorized yet; but I had a handle on how to direct her to intuitively search the refrigerator inventory. It never was a question of her learning the system. Rather it was my problem. I needed to get in tune with how much she could remember and recognize. It was I who had to learn the best way to teach Eve self-propelled lunch-making, with minimal involvement from me.

We continued to trip through the lunch-making routine together for the next few days. In a week or two, Eve was doing it on her own with varying success.

If I make the mistake of assuming that Eve can do any particular task—and she can't—that's my problem, not hers. My job is to accept the responsibility for failures and to correct my teaching method. When the successes do come, then the crown and title of Queen belong to Eve.

There was one more challenging aspect to lunchtime. Personally, I'm pretty sloppy about eating lunch on schedule. If someone makes a sandwich for me, I'll eat it. If not, I'll grab a convenient container of yogurt—and that's lunch. Or else, I'll skip it.

In her pre-aneurysm days, Eve's attention to the midday meal wasn't much better than mine.

Now, though, I considered a strict mealtime routine necessary for Eve's survival. She couldn't feel hunger "pangs." If something happened to me, Eve would need the added reinforcement of a schedule and a routine of eating nutritionally balanced meals. Therefore, it behooved me to invest my time in setting up a schedule for routine task management.

13

Rocking & Rolling the Daily Routine

At the early stage of Eve's recovery, I devoted several days to constructing an hour-by-hour daily task routine for her.

There were obvious benefits to habitualizing tasks. Eve always knew what she should do next. Whenever Eve's brain stuttered, she had a list for immediate reference. It limited the need to make choices, which could be exhausting and confusing—for both of us. It set up Eve for success and a feeling of accomplishment that I could reinforce, or reward at the end of the day. Plus, it freed up whole blocks of time for me to pursue my own interests. That freedom naturally enthused me.

When I announced the project to Eve, her response was less than enthusiastic; more like a "ho-hum." However, by the time I finished outlining the week, I felt inspired; not so much by the task schedule, but the way I planned to communicate the particulars with Eve.

Yes, we would get better together. I had written out the task schedule from her point of view—combined with mine. Because of my efforts to pick up on Eve's energy throughout the day, I had magically fallen into a rhythm. As I wrote (dum dee dee dum, dum dee doo wah) I felt I had captured a way Eve and I could dance through the day together, being carried by the varying levels of energy (the beat) from beginning to end.

I made each day a song with a rhythm and a melody. Let me explain. Think of any one of your favorite rock 'n' roll hits. Most songs start out stating the lyrical theme (breakfast); the beat begins and your toe starts tapping. Then comes the vocal (routine tasks), the hook that will keep you moving and grooving through the song. Next comes a riff of instrumental play (lunch), a moment to relax yet anticipate the return of the vocalist. The voice gets louder, more dramatic (interesting task), as it approaches the climax, the crescendo (cognitive exercise hour). Finally, the singer's voice fades (dinner). Nevertheless, the beat goes on, quieter now (gentle evening entertainment), but still playing in your head after the song has ended (bedtime).

I tuned into the beat of each varied day as I worked the tasks together with Eve. This made it easier for me to teach and easier for Eve to learn—to succeed—and feel deep-down that she had "accomplished" the day. Ta-dah!

Now that we were moving to the beat, we needed to get a melody, seven songs a week. Each day's melody sprang from a different theme: laundry on Monday (show tunes), living room on Tuesday (sambas), kitchen on Wednesday (Dixieland jazz), bathroom on Thursday (be-bop), her bedroom on Friday (the classics), joint projects such as shopping on Saturday (rock 'n' roll). Sunday was a day of rest, or outdoor projects in the summer, phone calls to friends, afternoon football or golf on TV, and something fun that eventually developed into the Eureka! adventures I describe later. Oh, yes. We'd also listen to our favorite CDs throughout the day.

Here's how those rhythms translated into a daily routine for Eve. Each day opened the same way. Eve made the coffee and fed the cats. Over coffee, she read our meditation for the day. I did my best to extract a motivation from the reading, to set a spiritual tone and promote a thoughtful consideration of the message. I'd express my gratitude for the coffee and give a voice to the cats, expressing their gratitude for the food.

Then we'd preview the day's tasks. Within each day the most complex projects were tackled in the morning; Lunch was a time for conversation, a review of the day, a shared, relaxing tea break, followed by a rejuvenating nap for Eve. Afternoon was the climactic final project (crescendos, if you will): the last of the laundry, the finishing touches for the rooms, easy mopping of the floors or Eve's favorite: vacuuming anything that resembled a rug or carpet.

Sometimes I could give her inherently interesting afternoon projects, such as tending the garden, writing a shopping list (in preparation for—gosh, golly, what fun—a trip to the supermarket), or helping me edit something I was writing to earn some money.

For the first few weeks, I worked hand-in-hand with Eve while we danced through the tasks that comprised her daily routine. I incorporated the "We will get better together" approach into my attitude. No, I didn't have to keep reminding myself. I began the regimen with a silent verbal request to my subconscious mind that I work through the day from Eve's point of view.

For example, Eve always sorted laundry by water temperature, often double-checking labels for laundry instructions. If that's what she did pre-aneurysm, I wasn't going to change it now.

This is an important aspect of the Eureka! strategy. My aim was to help Eve remember how to do things she had done in the past, not to teach her new methods. So a typical conversation with her might sound like, "Didn't you always put the hot whites through a second rinse?" Maybe her response would be to shift her weight on her feet as a signal that she wasn't certain, or she might stare at me blankly as if she couldn't remember or that she didn't comprehend the question. Or she might yawn to "say" she was bored or to indicate that the answer was, "Of course, dummy," or she might nod her head "yes." Whatever the response, I had a baseline on which to proceed as I gave more instructions and asked for a response.

We took hourly relaxation breaks, as I was learning to gauge her stamina, and the ebbs and flows of her energy through the day. The relaxation breaks were for me more than for Eve. Breaking down tasks into itty-bitty segments took concentration and monotonous repetition. The saving grace was that by the time I had learned a project from Eve's point of view, I had the steps memorized forever.

By slowing down my pace and working alongside of her, I had an opportunity to experience the nuances of her brain activity (or lack thereof). Let me explain. I soon learned that Eve's concept of "clean" was directly proportional to how much she liked cleaning the object. For instance, the shiny chrome kitchen sink was cleaned much more thoroughly than the tiny, lackluster bathroom sink. Eve had a difficult time matching the proper cleaning agent to a particular task's requirements. If she had her way, everything would be cleaned with a paper towel and a spray cleaner—even though she was reminded (by me) that for any particularly dirty job, a scouring pad would clean it faster, easier and better.

Eve didn't go in search of dirt to clean. If the daily routine didn't list "clean fingerprints on light switch plate," she would miss it no matter how many times I pointed it out. And yet, when it came to vacuuming, the frizzy ball in the corner didn't stand a chance. The furry cats ran for their lives. She interchanged her vacuum tools like a TV pitchman, demonstrating every product feature.

I had to rewrite the daily routine to include the details Eve always forgot, and asterisk the tasks requiring special cleaning products. Was this frustrating for the caregiver who disliked housecleaning more than Eve ever did? Oh, you betchya. However, I credit the "We will get better together" approach for helping me maintain some semblance of sanity and patience throughout the process. Obviously, the good Lord thinks I need frequent lessons in patience. I admit I am a slow learner. Somehow, every day I find the reason to learn how to correct my deficiencies—again.

As you can see, the daily routine is my battleground, my challenge, to raise my expectations for myself and to lower them for Eve. It's an opportunity to witness and participate in the seemingly nonlinear, illogical way a brain heals itself. On the days I can push my frustrations aside and align my subconscious with the challenges faced by Eve's brain, I reap enough rewards to fire my enthusiasm for the job.

SUGGESTION:

Take one of the most complicated routines that you would like the patient to relearn or remember. Depending on the patient's cognitive skill, break that task down into teachable parts. Be prepared to "show and tell," and don't hesitate to involve others in this process.

For example, if you want the patient to relearn omelet-making—and you don't know how to do it—ask someone else to teach it.

Hold off teaching anything "new" until after the patient has done the routine for a few weeks. You, of course, are the one who has to judge his/her problem-solving capabilities.

14

Enthusiasm–The Magic That Creates Eureka! Moments

I believe most educators agree that students pay more attention to, and learn best, those ideas and concepts that are taught using images and words that evoke an emotional response.

Being emotional is easy for me. Unfortunately, my initial response to most any surprising, disturbing, or even mildly disruptive positive event is generally negative. Though I hate to be bored, I dislike change. Now I don't want to waste any more words on psychoanalyzing myself on this subject. Obviously, my attitude is not healthy, and I've been trying to change me for years. Interestingly, if ever I was going to change—this was the moment. My motivation was strong to try whatever I could to rehabilitate Eve (and bring back my old boring life).

The way I saw it, Eve was so minimally motivated to return to what I considered a functioning human being, it would take all the emotional ammunition I could muster to effect that change. By nature, Eve was a positive person. I believed that the happier, more entertaining I could make life, the more apt she would be to pay attention, respond and, hopefully, learn. Time was of the essence. If happy emotions were good, then an enthusiastic approach would be even better.

Arrgh! One big question loomed over the household: How in the world could I pick myself up and be upbeat and enthusiastic in this situation?

My thoughts turned to memories of my mom, one of the most impossibly positive and enthusiastic people I have ever known. There was no such thing as a negative situation or crisis for my mom. She never seemed to be depressed, at least not around me. A "D" on my chemistry test, the loss of a job, the boyfriend who did not call—my mom taught me these were occasions to celebrate. According to Mom, here was an opportunity for the good Lord to prove that He never closes a door without opening a window. Every cloud has a silver lining. Every pile of poop signals that there's a pony nearby (or our cocker spaniel). So here in this caregiving situation was the opportunity for me to prove that at long last, I had become my mother's daughter. If she could make life into a never-ending game of triumphing over trouble and receiving "bad news" gratefully, so could I.

If that wasn't enough motivation to get me going, then I had another trick up my sleeve. I call it "How to instantly become everything I'm not." Yes, it's the ages-old self-con known as: "Act as if." I had practiced it on and off throughout my life, with more or less miraculous results. But this time the stakes were much higher than surviving a job loss. Yes, this time was like the last time I had to be reminded that I better "Act as if"—or else.

The scene was a 12-Step meeting many years ago. Truly, I was trying to save my life or, more precisely, to build a better one. Things weren't going so well. Granted, I had been sober for six months—which was good—but otherwise my life was a train wreck. I was out of work, out of money, out of friends. My sense of humor had vanished. Nothing was funny, including me. I was so depressed I could hardly talk without whimpering and whining.

One afternoon, after I had moaned about my plight for the umpteenth time in an A.A. meeting, a good-looking guy approached me. He was ten years my junior with three years of sobriety under his belt. I managed a smile. Perhaps my luck was finally changing?

"Hey, Madonna," he said. "I heard what you said in the meeting and I have a question for you."

Ah, hah, I thought. My wisdom is showing. Sure, laddy, bring on your question. I smiled and nodded.

He asked, "Tell me, aren't you sober about six months now?"

"Well, yes," I replied. "Why?"

"Because you sure don't sound like it," he retorted. "Seems to me that anyone who came in as far down the ladder as you did would be darned grateful that all of us have helped you to not pick up another drink today."

I was stunned. "B-but, I am grateful," I stuttered.

"Then why don't you show it by giving back to the beginners sitting around the table? You know, talk about how you're finally feeling happy, joyous and free."

"I don't feel very happy," I responded. "So why would I say that?"

"I suggest you 'act as if' and start sounding like you are in recovery." He continued, "Or else folks around here will start questioning whether you're grateful—or not." He flashed a smile, spun on his heel, and walked away.

I was dumbfounded. How dare that young punk speak to me that way? Then it hit me. Are the others talking about me? I had been around A.A. long enough to know that an ungrateful recovering alcoholic was someone to be pitied. Oh Lord, I didn't think I could handle being ostracized from A.A. I had failed on so many other counts.

Right then and there, I decided to change my ways. I shaped up. I dressed up. I pasted a smile on my face. At the next meeting, I faked it big time. Happy, joyous and free—that's me. I doubt anyone believed what I was saying, except (now don't laugh) me. For sure, it took a few weeks; but one day I noticed myself laughing at a joke. My depression began to lift. People invited me out for coffee. My sense of humor had returned.

Was it a miracle? You betchya. Just like the loaves and fishes. From a teeny-tiny ripple of effort came a gigantic wave of enthusiasm. It carried me for months, years. I never did get a big-time job again. But I did learn to be grateful for all the little ones I could put together to earn a decent living and recoup my self-respect. If I could do that back then, soggy brain and all, certainly I could try again for Eve, my friend, and for me, her clueless caregiver.

I had no idea what results to expect from our efforts. In a way, this was good. Unmet expectations can cause all sorts of emotional/psychological problems for the home caregiver. By feeding and fanning the flames of enthusiasm, the caregiver can leap over the hurdles of dwelling on unmet expectations and keep on going. One never knows when one might have a breakthrough. I'm sure medical science doesn't know everything about brain rehabilitation. So why should we caregivers assume that just because things aren't happening fast enough, there's no hope?

Here's how I learned that lesson the hard way, and mainly in retrospect. Thirty years ago my dad had a stroke. He was in the hospital for a few days and then he was home. He didn't come with instructions. Mom and I scoured the library for books to help us. There were none at all.

Dad's right side was temporarily paralyzed and remained weakened thereafter. The stroke robbed him of his sense of humor. Always a quiet man, he became quieter yet and profoundly depressed. My mother, brother and I tried to engage his mind with puzzles and games, which he dutifully played. We staged a game play every other night for a couple of months. Then we gave up. Everything was a chore.

The only time Dad appeared engaged was while watching his beloved Chicago Cubs and Bears sports teams on TV. Happy to see the light in his eyes for those baseball and football games, we let him be in front of the TV. After a while he was watching as many sports programs as he could—bowling, golf, and fishing. He became such a couch potato; it seemed he was in a stupor most of the time. We lost him mentally and emotionally. Physically, five years later he died of cancer.

I'm still kicking myself to this day. Three smart people in his family, all with boundless imaginations. You would think that one of us would be inspired to apply those talents to rehabbing Dad for longer than a couple of months.

So, why didn't we? Well, I, for one, was afraid of him. Not because he would ever hurt a flea; not because he was angry or mean. Perhaps I thought he would "break," like a fragile vase. Or maybe I thought I had no business invading his psyche and helping him to motivate himself.

But of this I'm certain. I am the one who needed help and courage. If anyone at all had suggested or encouraged me to use my imagination and go all out to create a rehab scenario based on Dad's love of sports, I would have done it in a heartbeat. I would have papered the walls with Chicago Bears logos. We would have played "catch" in the living room. Every night, we would have asked Dad to read aloud to all of us from Sports Illustrated. The family would have created Eureka! sports moments for Dad every day. If only someone had given us a hint that it could work!

I was determined not to let this happen to Eve. Never again did I want to say, "I should-of, could-of, would-of."

That's why over the years I have cultivated my enthusiasm for caregiving (and proved it to myself) by embellishing the routine with triggers to generate enthusiasm on Eve's behalf. When I sense Eve's apathy, our house becomes not a home, but a stage for a Broadway musical. I draw from Eve's lifelong love of the theater to help me help her be enthusiastic. I put a Broadway musical on the CD player, and it's showtime! Cue the actor (Eve) and stage crew (Eve, too). When the curtain opens on the living room scene, Eve has props (knickknacks) to dust, scenery (furniture) to rearrange and polish, set decoration (upholstery) to vacuum or fluff, lighting (lamps, windows, blinds) to clean and shine, and a script (not a written outline) to follow and check.

This is one metaphor I'm not afraid of extending beyond ridiculous limits. I use it to remind Eve of her good old days as a stage manager when, thanks to her skill and pride, she never missed a cue. Even if I simply employ the stage manager metaphor for comic relief, I believe I'm communicating the importance of her housekeeping role and encouraging her to take pride in her accomplishments.

In fact, it helps me communicate to Eve that I understand she'd rather be doing something more exciting than housework. I communicate that in her role as a homemaker, she is as deserving of applause as the stage manager is for her role in a play's success. Both are unsung heroes of the production and enthusiasm is the star of the show.

SUGGESTION:

Create your weekly routine of tasks for the patient (leaving one day for rest and fun). Work alongside the patient the first week so that you can get a handle on how the day feels to him or her—in terms of endurance, energy, and the ability to comprehend the task.

Review your patient's motivations and create a motivating scenario, when and where it is needed. Here are some examples: administering an office, captaining a sailboat, planning a family reunion, painting a picture, creating a patchwork quilt, coaching a sports team, etc.

If the patient is employed and able to work, much of your motivational factor is already provided. If it's a real motivator for the patient, extend the metaphor to include household chores.

Meanwhile, you can be practicing "acting as if" you are enthusiastic about the daily routine by initiating a reward system for a job well done. Praise the patient often; and pause before you criticize mistakes. Always question if errors are the patient's fault—or if the problem just might be the way the task was taught.

15

Power Plays and Other Struggles

I didn't need to be a rocket scientist to notice that Eve was more highly motivated to perform some tasks better than others. Her favorites were: making morning coffee, fixing dinners, going grocery shopping (which eventually included driving the car, a motivator in itself), doing laundry (go figure) and—ta-dah!—vacuuming the floors, walls, furniture and ceilings.

However, we had knockdown, drag out fights over her reluctance to actually plan meals for the week, write shopping lists, follow the shopping lists, dusting, scrubbing the tub, monitoring the refrigerator inventory, and finding/cleaning dirt in the corners. Most of these (ahem) spirited discussions are still taking place, as they have over the past seven years.

Oh no, you say. Oh yes. I'm sorry if I led you to fantasize that at some point Eve and I strolled off into the rainbow-gated land of happily ever after. But previously I mentioned that I believed Eve still needed daily attention, lest she give in to impulsive, compulsive behaviors that would cloud her mind and eventually unravel the daily routine.

Even though my outlook on our mutual recovery from her brain aneurysm is "We will get better together," it isn't always viewed that way by Eve. It's not that she doesn't "get it" most of the time. She does. However, when her mind is fuzzy, especially when she's low on energy or just physically tired, she forgets.

Then my first reaction is to tell her what to do next. Even if that direction is simply "Isn't it time for your nap?" I have assumed a power role—Queen Caregiver—in a relationship that is supposed to be equal partners. This is not good; I am undermining my own "We will get better together" strategy.

I can see why I bark orders at Eve. I know that oftentimes when Eve fails to accomplish a task, I'm visited by fear. I fear that Eve is showing signs of dreaded dementia, or something else that can debilitate a recovering brain that's been battered and bashed by strokes and seizures.

But the problem is mine, not Eve's. I have to calm down. I have to teach myself that Eve's fate is beyond my control. My job is to be there on a daily basis to help, with no expectations.

Handling my fear is important to Eve's recovery, as well as my serenity. Here's why: The intuitive communicative process flows and goes both ways. Since we are operating most days on a sub-conscious, emotional level, Eve can tune into my fears. Whether she thinks about it or not, she perceives at some level that there is a power imbalance and she is suddenly in control.

When I bark an order at her out of fear, she resents it. The stroke has weakened her ability to deal with that resentment maturely. She is going to jab back at me somehow.

Meanwhile, ever since the brain aneurysm, Eve is more prone to seeking instant gratification through obsessive/compulsive behaviors, such as Internet solitaire and reading nonsense. (Keep in mind that Eve has also previously overcome addiction. Though she has recovered, and those addictive tendencies have diminished, they have never gone away.) She knows intuitively that her obsessive behaviors not only aggravate me, but cause me fear. However, when she's in the middle of a power play, her feelings of power-lessness (over her brain disabilities) rise to the surface. She will get back at me if for no other reason than to feel more in control.

I don't know how to cure power imbalances overnight. I do

know that honesty (with myself and Eve) helps stabilize the power in the relationship.

Rather than going through the day apologizing, I would prefer to set up scenarios where either one of us can tell the other one she is getting too big for her britches. Unfortunately, that sort of face-to-face self-appraisal is not part of Eve's "old" spirit and personality. Using the "We will get better together" approach, I have to let her know that I know when I've gone beyond my boundaries and invaded her territory—her right to be her own person even when her behavior is wrong. For my well-being, I need to call a spade a spade. I do have a right to be me.

It's truly a high-wire act for any caregiver. It calls for lots of humility (certainly not my strongest suit). But if I keep in mind that this, too, will help Eve recover and help me maintain my serenity, then I'm motivated to try. Trying counts. Eve can perceive that, too.

So I decided to include an honesty review of sorts in the daily routine. It became an integral aspect of our morning meditation session. Each day, I communicated with Eve that I understood her tendency to compulsively play on the computer or to read in lieu of doing housework. I would explain that my fear was (is) that such behavior would lead to sloppy, fuzzy thinking and an inability to automatically function at a survival level (if something happened to me). I further acknowledged that there was scientific evidence she was more prone to developing dementia because of the aneurysm. I would tell her that I feared seeing the signs of dementia and I wished she would fear it too. Maybe then she would fight her desires for instant gratification.

I also learned a couple of tricks from A.A. sponsorship. One such technique is to allow the behavior to continue until the patient has experienced the adverse consequences and feels the emotional pain of regret. For example, I might allow Eve to play on the computer through dinnertime; then let her deal with eating late alone. This tactic calls for careful judgment on the part of the caregiver. Obviously, you don't want the patient to endanger anyone's safety.

The other technique is to require the patient to perform the obsessive behavior every hour for ten minutes. Often, this takes all the "fun" out of doing the aggravating behavior.

There are many combinations of the power play equation. All come with payoffs for both parties. Often, the balance of power switches back and forth with lightning speed. Without mutual acknowledgement that a power struggle exists, chances are the struggle will continue. But when all the cards are placed face up on the table, more often than not the struggle dissolves. Winning is no longer "fun" for either party. I believe that even a cognitively impaired patient can sense that the game's over at a subconscious level. But it will never happen unless one of the two—meaning the caregiver—calls the hand.

SUGGESTION:

It might seem difficult to believe that the disabled patient is bullying the caregiver, but it happens.

A caregiver who feels like a victim might need outside help from a professional to help balance the power. I certainly did. I didn't want to be a victim; nor did I want to be an emotional bully. On more than one occasion, I spoke to counselors about the balance of power. Counseling with a psychological therapist, social worker, life coach, trained religious counselor, or a wise friend or family member might help.

Don't wait on this one. Call today.

16

Evolution of Eureka!

I did not invent the Eureka! memories and motivation strategy. Rather, it slowly evolved from my efforts to bring back the old Eve one day at a time. It was a reactionary versus an anticipatory process. I didn't know what was going to come next—good or bad. Rehabilitating Eve's initial disabilities was a "one step backward and two steps forward" process. I would think I had solved one problem only to have a hidden one revealed. As Eve got better, some new ones popped up, such as those always challenging obsessive/compulsive behaviors.

Looking back, I can see the Eureka! strategy began unfolding while Eve was lying comatose in the hospital. At that time, I was acting intuitively to emotionally communicate with her on a subconscious level. I did not consciously have a clue as to what I was doing until the day Eve entertained friends who had made the long drive up from Chicago to visit her. When they entered the room, I left to take a break. When I returned, I stopped in the doorway and listened. It was like waiting for popcorn to pop in the microwave. Every few moments, one or the other visitor would shout at my comatose friend, "Eve, wake up." Sometimes they shouted in unison.

I smiled to myself, not because I thought there was anything very funny about this sad scenario. What amused me was a thought that kept dancing in my head: Eve will never, ever come out of that coma as long as the two of you are shouting at her. It's a futile effort. Can't you see she's hiding from you? Eve's playing a game.

What in the world would possess me to have such a thought? Well, it could have been triggered by seeing a faint coy smile on Eve's lips. I would swear it wasn't there before I left the room. Was this my admittedly overactive imagination in action? Or did I intuitively perceive a playful game of hide-and-seek? I'll never know for sure.

But after that visitation, I began developing my own personal strategy for trying to bring back Eve. I wouldn't waste my breath trying to rouse her from the coma if it looked like she was deep in "sleep." No, I'd wait for the moment she'd shift her position, or cough, and then I'd go at her, blasting away with both barrels.

Amazingly, much of the time, it worked. Eve would open up her eyes for a few moments. Then her eyelids would flutter as if to say "hi." For the moments she was "awake," I'd go over the top with a joyful greeting and deliver a teaser message: "If you'll stay awake longer, I've got a great story to tell you." Often I perceived a struggle on Eve's part to stay conscious. If and when that happened, I'd tell her the latest news or gossip as fast as I could to reward her efforts.

I used this same technique weeks later when the still-comatose Eve was in the nursing home. I'd ask a nurses' aide to help me strap her in a wheelchair and I'd wheel my unconscious friend to their cheery garden room with a TV. For the next 15 minutes or so, I'd treat Eve to a little play-by-play football action, courtesy of the Green Bay Packers Sunday telecast. Generally, Eve would "come out" of her coma to see a dramatic play (cued by the TV announcers' excited voices or mine). Sometimes she'd awaken for several minutes before she would slip away again. It was a highlight of the week.

This is the stuff Eureka! memories are made of. The process is different from other textbook-style cognitive or memory-recall exercises. Eureka! happens most often when the patient is involved in an emotionally stimulating, creative process. For this purpose, I define the creative process as participating in a social activity, playing sports or a game, music-making, treasure hunting (shopping) or crafting a work of art. Highly emotional conversation qualifies as Eureka! when it involves joke-telling, brainstorming solutions to problems, or thoughtfully discussing personal wishes or needs. Crossword puzzles or jigsaw puzzle-solving become Eureka! when a high-energy person works with the patient.

The Eureka! triggering mechanism is activated by an activity that has high emotional impact for the patient. In the act of being "creative," the door is opened to the subconscious mind, because the conscious, logical mind steps aside to allow the subconscious mind free rein. In other words, it's playtime!

As we know, the subconscious is where all the high-impact memories (mostly from long ago) are stored. The memories are linked to each other. Their content includes the behaviors and input from the five senses that were happening at the time the memory was made. All of this is linked and categorized by emotion. The Eureka! memory strategy magically brings back those powerful memories—and all of that wonderful content we caregivers want to retrieve such as pre-brain-injury behaviors.

Following are three examples of how the Eureka! strategy evolved. If I hadn't been paying attention, I might never have noticed the recovery "miracles" that were happening.

Throughout Eve's third year of recovery, she slowly progressed. As the holidays approached, she was anticipating an end-of-year birthday bash with her lifelong Chicago buddies. All of them had just turned sixty years old and they wanted to celebrate by doing their hometown in style over the Christmas holiday.

I drove Eve down to Chicago from our northeast Wisconsin home. I was celebrating, too. It was my first real break from daily caregiving since Eve's stint in the inpatient rehabilitation hospital.

When Eve came home after her reunion, I quizzed her on the week. Thanks to phone calls from her friends, I already knew about their excursions to museums, the Magnificent Mile and various chi-chi restaurants. Good thing I heard the reports because Eve's recall of her ventures was sketchy. One of her friends (who had been Eve's maid of honor) had videotaped a walk down memory lane that the three of them had taken one evening after dinner. At first, I could barely stand to watch the tape.

As the threesome sat on a couch, Eve's friends took turns trying to jolt her memory. Could Eve remember Sister Mary Knuckle Cracker, the fifth-grade nun who wielded a wooden ruler like a sword? How about their drive to the beach in Eve's first car, a shiny red convertible? Remember dancing the polka at Stash Przybylo's wedding?

On and on, Eve's friends chatted while she sat like a lump on a log, looking bewildered—or even worse, giggling instead of responding to their questions and prompts. And then her friends burst into a favorite song from their school days, "Carmen Carmella." At first, Eve was speechless; then there was a spark. She joined in the chorus, singing "when bells are ringing." She couldn't remember all the words; but you could hear her loud and clear on the words she did.

The videotape demonstrated what I was just beginning to understand. Eureka! was triggered here because Eve had been totally immersed in a creative process, the singing of the old favorite song. In fact, I'd say Eureka! touched all three of them. Bouncing and giggling, they all looked like carefree sixth-graders (with wrinkles) at a glee club rehearsal. In the act of going to that "creative" place in her mind (however feeble her attempt), Eve was opening the door to her subconscious mind. That's where all those high-impact, youthful, emotional memories linked to concurrent preteen behaviors were stored. They had been sitting there for decades waiting to be tapped by the "today" Eureka! memory of enthusiastic, emotional song singing.

The jury is still out on whether or not I really wanted to bring back the clowning antics of a sixth-grader. On the other hand, that behavior was also linked to the lifelong bond of friendship among that group of friends. I did want Eve to be touched by all those feelings associated with that friendship.

The recall process works better when all (or most) of the five senses—sight, touch, hearing, smell, taste—are involved in the present day Eureka! memory-making moment. Most importantly, the more enthusiasm and emotion generated by the caregiver (or group), the better it is for creating the high-impact, emotional Eureka! trigger memory that links to those past memories, behaviors and emotions we want to revive.

It is not necessary for the patient to be able to consciously recall the memory. Eureka! happens whether or not the initial memory-making event is actually "remembered." This is how Eve's emotions—which she was not able to consciously recall—came back anyway.

Here is an example of how Eureka! works to the benefit of both patient and caregiver. Soon after the holiday break, I began writing the outline for my book, *Brain, Heal Thyself*. It became my New Year's resolution. I reworked Eve's daily routine so that she could devote her afternoons to typing it (a task I disliked, but that Eve welcomed as an interesting diversion from housework.) On some level, Eve perceived this as a way to help me succeed in my career, in the spirit of "We will get better together."

Eve was doing a good job. Alas, I couldn't say the same for me. The problem of writing a memoir about Eve's recovery was hampered by a simple fact: I hadn't taken any notes. How was I going to remember the events well enough to write 50,000 words on the subject? I had written detailed outlines of the first three chapters but uh, duh—what happened next?

I was scratching my head and doodling on the blank page when Eve came into the room, proudly carrying the three typed chapters. She smiled as she handed them to me, and then sat down. The expectant look on her face said she was eager to do more typing. I had nothing to give her. And then I had an idea. In retrospect, it was one of my best.

"Why don't you read what I wrote back to me," I said to her. She shrugged an "okay." At first timid, Eve's voice grew stronger and more expressive as she read the pages.

Something incredible happened then. As I listened to her reading, I got in sync with the rhythm. Somehow that rhythm inspired me to remember events. I interrupted Eve, saying things like, "Write this down, Eve. I remember you were able to recall the name of your college immediately following the first brain surgery." It was an integral part of the story I had forgotten. Eve continued reading. I continued remembering, stopping her to make a note. At the subconscious level, we were writing the book together.

Now I know Eve couldn't consciously help me remember the events as I was recounting them. She was in a coma for three months. However, I believe that the events experienced by Eve were recorded in her subconscious mind. Was Eve conveying her misty memories while she was reading to me? Was she giving me subtle clues through shifts in her body energy? Or inflections in her voice? Or in her body language? All I know is that her presence triggered my recall of the *Brain, Heal Thyself* experience. I could intuitively feel it.

At some point, this Eureka! adventure in book writing became a motivator in and of itself. In other words, it took on a life of its own. For Eve, it became something to anticipate and to pay attention to. It helped her feel as though she had a handle on the four months she had lost, memory-wise. It even triggered a fleeting memory or two from those lost months that previously she could not recall. On a subconscious level, Eve was helping to create a Eureka! moment with her contributions to the creation of the book. Plus, she was helping me do something I wanted to accomplish. That made the "book moment" memorable.

Here's another aspect of the Eureka! strategy that makes it different from most ordinary memory rehabilitation routines. Eureka! involves two people (who care about each other) sharing emotional energy, having fun, experiencing life, and creating something— together. Both are making an emotional investment with an expected positive outcome for both. It's not a teaching experience where one has the "power" and the other doesn't; but it can be a learning experience where both participants come away having been taught a lesson.

I recall one weekend when the flusher-thingy on our toilet broke. To hear my cry of dismay, you'd think the bathroom had flooded. I am not mechanical. Fixing toilets had been Eve's department pre-aneurysm. I gave Eve the bad news and then proceeded to search for the plumber's phone number.

"Why don't you go to Walmart, pick up the part and fix it yourself," Eve suggested.

"You've got to be kidding," I replied. "I don't know anything about toilet repair. That's why God invented plumbers. But hey, did you ever replace a flusher?"

"I think I did a long time ago." Eve cautiously added, "I'm not sure I remember how to do it."

Bingo! Here was a great Eureka! adventure, whether I wanted it or not.

We toddled off to Walmart together. We searched out the toilet parts display, where we debated the two choices: plastic or metal. I opted for the cheaper one, fully expecting that we'd end up calling a plumber in the end.

When we got back to the house and the bathroom, I lifted the tank lid. As I stared into the murky depths, I turned to Eve and said, "You do it. It looks too scary, too complicated for me. I'll read the instructions to you." Eve shrugged and rolled up her sleeves. I had barely gotten to Step Two when Eve announced, "I'm done. Let's try it." She flushed the toilet as I held my breath. It worked.

"You did it," I shouted. I didn't have to fake my enthusiasm—it was boundless. "Eureka! You fixed it. Hallelujah! Let's have some ice cream to celebrate. You saved us big money."

Later in the week I found Eve sitting on the utility room floor among parts from our broken vacuum cleaner. (We had two.)

"What are you doing?" I asked her.

"Oh, just replacing a broken belt."

"How did you know it was the belt? That vacuum's been broken for months."

"I don't know," Eve said. "I guess I just knew it."

"And where did you get a new belt?" I asked.

She replied, "While I was out for my walk yesterday, I decided to stop at the appliance repair shop to get more vacuum bags. Then I thought of the belt and bought that, too."

I was baffled. That vacuum had been hiding in the back of the closet forever. I had told Eve to use the other one until I got around to taking this one in for repair. I don't know what made her remember where the vacuum cleaner was stored, then realize it was a broken belt, then figure out how to replace it. I have to presume the toilet triumph triggered that area of her brain. Goodbye, Mr. Handyman. The "old" Eve—Miss Fixit of the past—is back. Eureka!

SUGGESTION:

It's time to start creating your own unique style of Eureka! Make yourself a cup of tea, grab a note pad, sit back and relax.

Think back to the good times you've most recently shared with the patient, before or after the stroke or brain trauma. Pick two events. In a few words, write about what made them fun for you and guess (or ask) what made them fun for the patient.

Did the events or people involved have anything to do with the patient's lifelong motivations? Guess or ask the patient.

Can you duplicate the circumstances in any way (same place, same people, same activity)?

If there's a possibility you can use this information to create an activity, then file your note in your new Eureka! idea file, drawer or shoebox for the future.

17

How Eureka! Feels

With all this talk about enthusiasm and the ability to evoke high-impact emotional reactions, you might be thinking I'm some sort of superwoman caregiver.

I am not. Actually, I am generally quiet and not very outgoing. I admit I have emotions; however, they often tend to be negative. To me, the glass is half-empty rather than half-full.

In other words, I've had to work at changing me for the sake of establishing a positive recovery environment for Eve's brain and to control my fears, frustration and stress. This would be very hard work indeed, if it wasn't for that wonderful self-con technique of "acting as if."

Whenever my intuition tells me that it's time to inject Eureka! into our lives, I remember my mom. Then I pretend (act as if) I inherited her marvelous talent to make everyday Eureka! for her family.

My mom had that special super-energy that made dull parties come alive and made heads turn when she strolled into a restaurant, church meeting or the grocery store. On many a childhood shopping trip with Mom, I would be dumbfounded as complete strangers would walk up to her and start talking as if she was a long-lost friend. As best I could ever tell, the strangers were attracted to her warm, enthusiastic energy, a responsive spark in her eyes and her apparent interest in whatever they had to say.

Perhaps you've known a person like my mom in your life. If so, you might conjure up an image of your special person, while I relate the story of how Mom turned another ordinary weekday dinner into a Eureka! memory for me. (Look for the similarities between my mom and you and your special person. That way you might actually feel how Eureka! can make an emotional impact in your life and the patient's.)

Throughout my childhood Mom worked as a teller at the neighborhood bank. I was ten years old and my brother was seven when this anecdote happened. It took place during dinner, which was usually the Eureka! memory-making hour of power in our house. The family was seated around the kitchen table. Mom said to Dad, "You'll never believe the bizarre thing that happened at work today."

Yes, he would. Hardly a dinner passed that Mom didn't have a happy, sad, funny or weird anecdote to report over dessert. Her little stories were always more entertaining than whatever was on TV. We were all ears to hear "the latest."

Here's how I remember her story. It was noon and she was eating alone in the bank's lunchroom when in walked Bob, the cocky young teller they just hired, and Mabel, the grouchy receptionist.

Between bites of his salami sandwich, Bob asked Mom for a suggestion on good children's books to read to his toddler.

"Oh, I have several favorites," Mom said. "My kids always loved *Billy Goat's Gruff*, *Uncle Wiggly*, and my all-time favorite, *Little Black Sambo*.

"I don't remember *Little Black Sambo*," grunted grouchy Mabel. "I never heard of it," piped up Bob. Mom swallowed her sandwich bite and smiled. "Well then, let me tell you the story."

And so she did. She had memorized *Little Black Sambo* after a thousand readings to us kids. Within a minute, Bob and Mabel had stopped eating. They were mesmerized. Mom continued. Word quickly spread throughout the bank that there was "live" entertainment in the lunchroom. Two more tellers and a loan officer came in and sat down at the table. The vice-president of the bank poked his head in the door. The bank president pushed past him to get a seat at the table. How he loved to listen to Mom's stories.

"And so Sambo watched from the tree as the tiger ran around the trunk—faster and faster and faster yet. G-r-r-r! Then, before Sambo's eyes, the frenzied tiger whipped himself into butter. Sambo was saved!"

The lunchroom erupted into applause. Mom bowed.

To this day, what totally fascinates me about this story is that I can remember what we had for dinner—meatloaf—and that I felt so warm and safe looking out the window at the snowy cold winter night. I remember Mom's amused smile signaled the end of the story. My dad chuckled and my dorky little brother laughed. (He didn't get it.) I was totally impressed, in awe of my mom again.

How weird, how zany, how entertaining can you get? That's Eureka! in action. Simple, powerful, emotional and surprising. Just a little to the left of the expected. A little bit over the top. But always and forever memorable.

No, I'll never forget Mom's simple little story from a half-century ago about the day the bank stood still while Mom told a children's bedtime story to the bank employees at lunch. And I'll never forget what we had for dessert that night—Del Monte fruit cocktail (everyone got a cherry).

To this day, whenever I see a children's book, enter a dark and solemn bank, open a container of whipped butter, taste Mom's meatloaf or I'm forced to eat canned fruit cocktail, Eureka! is triggered. I am instantly transported back to a time when I felt warm, cozy, safe, loved and always entertained.

That's what Eureka! can do for you and the patient together. The Eureka! strategy works by making an emotional connection between today's creative, enthusiastic activities and adventure, and yesterday's high-impact emotional memories, and all similar linked memories in-between.

In the process, Eureka! triggers the behaviors and feelings associated with that initial memory. Hence, the patient is stimulated to remember how he or she used to be, before the stroke or brain trauma. It's a different approach to home rehabilitation—based on remembering—not teaching something new or different.

Oh, now I'm on a roll with remembering my own personal Eureka! feeling. Have you recalled a Eureka! person from your past life yet? It really helps show you the way.

Here's another short anecdote that shows how Eureka! can influence behavior. Back again to my younger years, when I was a typical preteen with a messy bedroom. As usual, Saturday was room-cleaning day. Around noon, one of my friends phoned, and I escaped the house before Mom had a chance to check my claim that my room was clean. I played all afternoon. When I returned home, I learned that Mom had declared my room an official "Disaster Area." At least that's what Mom had scrawled on a sign that was taped to my bedroom door. She had taken the time to draw an official-looking seal at the bottom. Tentatively, I turned the doorknob, halfway hoping that Mom had cleaned my room while I was gone.

No such luck. Instead, Mom had taped little notes to each and every fuzzball that festooned the hardwood bedroom floor. One fuzzball post said, "Help me. I've been marooned under the bed for five months." Another said, "I have a date with the garbage can." And on it went: "Please help me, I'm getting fatter"; "Did you see my mommy anywhere?"; "Can I join my friends under the desk?" etc. It must have taken Mom forever to label all the wayward fuzzballs in my room.

I started to laugh and I continued to giggle as I cleaned up my mess for the next hour. It was almost as much fun as finding Easter eggs. My mother never had to tell me again to dust mop my room. Really, it was too much fun to ever again call it a chore.

If there's one housework chore I enjoy nowadays, it's dust-mopping the hardwood floors. It's like a family reunion. I'm sure I'm living with the grandkids from my original fuzzball memory.

Knowing how Eureka! happened in my life helps me intuitively recognize when Eve needs a boost of creativity or enthusiasm in her day.

SUGGESTION:

Remember the Eureka! memory-makers in your life. Think of one or two otherwise ordinary occasions that they made memorable. How? Why?

If that person is alive, call him or her for a chat. Perhaps that conversation will trigger more ideas on how you can recognize Eureka! opportunities for you and the patient.

If that person is in heaven, ask him or her to be an angel and give you some help.

18

Recognizing Eureka! Every Day

Good news! Many ordinary, everyday activities have Eureka! potential. The trick is to recognize the emotion-evoking opportunities. Then we can maximize the Eureka! effect and use that emotional memory recall to help bring back lost skills and behaviors.

During Eve's early recovery, I thought many of her leaps were purely miraculous. One day a chance comment from a friend about the nature of miracles made me stop and think twice. Perhaps Eve's improvement isn't totally due to miracles. Maybe it's the result of something I did.

Well, gosh darn, leave it to the Almighty to toss the ball back in my lap. If I did something that helped Eve, then I had to figure out what that was. And then I would have to figure out a way to repeat what I did. That sounds a lot like work to me. It is; but it can also be rewarding and fun, too.

Following are several examples of how Eureka! mostly happened to us—and how I slowly learned to recognize what was happening to Eve.

RETRIEVING COGNITIVE SKILLS

Even in early recovery, it appeared Eve was reading books and magazines at her usual pre-aneurysm pace, judging from the speed of her page turning. However, if I stopped her and asked her what she had just read, she couldn't give me an intelligent summary.

For example, if I stopped her in the middle of a novel, such as *Gone with the Wind*, and asked her what was happening at that point, she'd typically respond, "I'm reading *Gone with the Wind*. It's about Scarlett O'Hara's life on the plantation." She sounded like a 5th grader giving a book report.

Did Eve not comprehend what she was reading, or did she not understand my question, or could she not express an answer? I begged her to write one-paragraph book reports; but she wouldn't or couldn't do it. I assumed she could comprehend what she was reading, or she would never finish the 300-page books she was reading. I also assumed she could hold the memory of the plot in her head from day to day. But why couldn't Eve convey what she comprehended to me?

Every day I'd try a new approach; but as time went on I felt like I did the first time my grandpa presented the "chicken or the egg" conundrum to my juvenile brain. I spent hours trying to solve an unsolvable puzzle.

I borrowed some children's books from the library, with the idea that we would return to the basic mechanics of reading and comprehension. I made this mistake only once. Eve read two pages of the grammar school reader, stopped, closed the book with a sigh and delivered one of those "Don't ever insult me like this again" dirty looks.

I didn't; but I didn't give up trying, either.

Somewhere along the line, a friend gave Eve the book, *Crosswords for Dummies*. It was aptly named. I had tried a couple of the puzzles and, gosh darn, I couldn't do them. But I knew they would have been a snap for the "old" Eve to solve. Perhaps the two of us could work a crossword puzzle during her cognitive play hour.

In the beginning, Eve couldn't or wouldn't do the puzzles by herself. So I, the world's worst crossword-puzzle-solver, had to help her. This was a challenge. Eve would stare blankly at the clue. I'd tell her to read it to me. I'd ask her to count spaces and tell me how many letters were needed. Then she'd look at me expectantly and I'd look at her blankly. We'd both shrug and go on to the next clue. After twenty minutes, our puzzle would be pimpled with erasures. On a rare occasion, I actually came up with a word that fit. Naturally, I'd be extremely proud of myself and Eve would congratulate me. We'd continue until I gave up after an hour. This was not very therapeutic for Eve; it was just plain sad for me.

Because our options were so limited, I didn't want to quit trying to make a game of it. I figured if Eve had done crosswords in the past, she could remember how to do them again. After a week of failures, I invented another approach to solving the puzzle.

This time I asked Eve to read a clue, and I would give her additional clues. It stretched my vocabulary recall to the limits; but that's why God invented dictionaries. My main goal was to have Eve successfully guess the word. I'd give her sentences using a synonym or opposite word. I'd do pantomimes. I'd create an imaginary scenario which might involve the word. ("The computer is sick because it has a five–letter word.") Of course, I had no idea what the answer was either. Even if the answers were at the back of the book, I wouldn't dare look at them. I would be telling Eve that "cheating" was okay. It wasn't. So I spent the hour guessing. It was like the blind leading the blind. However, I did have Eve's attention.

Amazingly, something about the process (of me making a fool of myself) spurred Eve to take the reins. Somewhere deep inside I believe she recognized that she was better at the game than I. She felt so sorry for my plight that she was motivated to help me by coming up with the right word—thus putting an end to my agony—in the spirit of "We will get better together."

It took a couple of years of this convoluted crossword play before the blessed moment came when Eve finally said, "Do you mind if I work the puzzle by myself today?" Hey, Eve, what's a four-letter word for Eureka!?

Truthfully, I was a little sad to see this era in "We" cognitive therapy come to an end. How often does life offer an opportunity to witness such miraculous progress—a reversal of roles in cognitive therapy? I understand that most professional therapists cannot devote the time to creating a setting where the patient rises to the occasion to help the therapists. But they certainly could take some time to teach the caregiver how to do it at home. Helping the patient take the lead in puzzle-solving is an ideal strategy for empowering the patient and giving them the motivating taste of success.

This strategy can be applied to any activity where the patient had previously taken the lead and which now must be done by the "inept" caregiver. I truly believe that my incompetence at crossword-puzzle-solving, my so-so cooking capabilities and my pitiful attempts to fix household mechanical or electrical problems motivated Eve to try and try again, until it came back to her—like magic.

RETRIEVING COMMUNICATION SKILLS

During the early months of Eve's recovery, her attention span during conversations was minimal. Her eyes would glaze over and she would yawn three minutes into any discussion. Granted, most of our conversations were monotonous monologues delivered by me; so her boredom was understandable.

I tried to engage her in discussions after the evening news hour on TV; but even politics and show business gossip (topics she relished discussing in the past) drew no comment when I addressed them.

Talk about resistance! The more I tried to entice Eve to comment on current events, the less she did it. Every day presented a new opportunity for me to practice patience in the face of passive-aggressive behavior. I had to figure out how to persuade Eve that talking with me was an opportunity to help herself. Progress was slow in coming.

Interestingly, I had begun to solve the problem months before; but I hadn't realized it. One morning, as I was practicing my relaxation routine, I was blessed with an insight. (Another benefit of being relaxed—that's the time ah-ha insights come to visit.) As usual, I was reading one of my favorite passages from the Emmett Fox book of daily meditations. Eve was busily recording her one-sentence summary of a 12-Step book's thought for the day. Momentarily, I was gripped by nostalgia as I recalled a spirited conversation Eve and I had engaged in many years before, over how Emmett's lesson *du jour* applied to a situation in our lives. I missed having those discussions. On an impulse, I handed my book to Eve and said, "Read this Emmett Fox meditation aloud to me. Then we'll discuss it."

I noticed a shift in her position; she puffed up, her energy swelled as if I had invited her on stage. She articulated the words, intelligently and expressively, with inflections and dramatic pauses in all the right places. No doubt in my mind that Eve understood what she was reading.

I asked her to summarize what she had just read. At first, she stuttered. I asked her to write a one-sentence summary. I waited for her to do it, then I asked her to read it. She had written, "This was Emmett's story about the 'golden key'." Well, that was true—albeit brief. I questioned her again. "Isn't this about a person turning over a difficult situation to God, going about his business without thinking about the problem and, in the end, somehow the problem is solved without the person's interference or help?"

Eve nodded. "Say yes," I pleaded. She did. "And now tell me the lesson of the reading in your own words."

Slowly, the words came out of her mouth. "If I'm worried about something, God will take care of it."

Well, that's closer to the meaning than her previous summary.

"Eve, can you give me a recent example of how you turned something over?"

Eve looked thoughtful. Five minutes passed. "Well?" I finally interrupted the silence.

"Well, what?" she asked.

Oh, rats, I thought. I was frustrated now. What could I do?

I decided not to push her any further. At least she had related the gist of the message to herself. For now, I still was not sure what to change. She was closer to being correct, but so far away from being the spirited Eve of old.

As the message in the meditation directed, I decided to "turn it over" and go about my business that day. As the days went on, I would ask Eve to read the meditations in the morning and write her summaries. Then we would devote five minutes to discussing how to apply the spiritual message we had just learned to the day ahead, even if I was doing most of the discussing with myself. Day after day, I dragged Eve down all the mental paths we used to explore together. Initially, I would pose questions and then answer them myself. As time went on, I began asking Eve for more precise or thoughtful contributions. I don't know how many months it took before my animated "monologue-dialogues" became real discussions.

What I do know is that I sat down with Eve each morning with minimal expectations for her performance and big expectations for my patience. I also told Eve that this was our daily A.A. meeting, thereby reinforcing the basic "We will get better together" motivation. Eventually, I believe that her subconscious sense of responsibility took over and she realized that she had a role in helping me to stay sober and sane, too. In order to do that, she had to talk and I had to listen.

Motivation-wise, at the subconscious level, I was reinforcing our longtime pact we had made years before. It was a commitment. We both knew that without sobriety there could be no friendship. Fortunately for us, the "We will get better together" motivational strategy is an integral part of the 12-Step program sponsorship practice.

RETRIEVING SOCIAL SKILLS

At some point it occurred to me that perhaps Eve needed more of a challenge than helping me stay sober and sane. Yes, I did need daily reinforcement; but I had ways of obtaining this without requiring Eve's help. Eve knew this, at least on a subconscious level. Perhaps helping me wasn't a big enough challenge for her. Maybe she needed to start attending meetings again, so she could see beginners struggling to learn what she knew deep inside. Maybe the action of helping others would help Eve regain some of that social, emotional spark for her spirit.

As the days progressed, I became more confident that the "We will get better together" approach was the key to helping me recognize the opportunities for social-emotional recovery within our ordinary lives. Interestingly, I discovered that I didn't have to be part of the "we" equation. I could enlist the aid of friends and even strangers.

When Eve began attending 12-Step meetings again, the local women's group welcomed her with understanding and kindness. When it was Eve's turn to speak at these meetings, the women patiently listened as Eve frequently paused and rambled in her attempts to contribute to the group discussion. Sometimes she did not address the subject, or she forgot what she was saying midsentence. As the months progressed, Eve relearned to talk coherently on topic. As she gained confidence in herself and trusted her acceptance by the group, Eve could devote more attention to listening and relating to the others, especially those who had problems. It was a happy day indeed when I heard Eve say to one frightened newcomer, "I know how you feel. I remember when I worried about attending my first wedding celebration in sobriety. I suggest you take your sponsor's phone number with you, so you can call her before you get in trouble. I'll give you my number. You can call me, too."

I could hardly believe what I was hearing. Eve had reassumed her responsibilities as a veteran of the 12-Step program. She had also made two mini-leaps in brain recovery. Cognitively speaking,

Eve had perceived someone else's problem, remembered her own experience from the long-ago past and couched her words in the traditional 12-Step format of offering a suggested action. On the emotional/social level, Eve had applied the "We will get better together" strategy to help somebody else in emotional distress.

RETRIEVING PHYSICAL SKILLS

While Eve was relearning how to perform household tasks, I was trying to establish the rhythm within the day. Over time, I realized that we regularly encountered several roadblocks on our daily journey to happy routine. In addition to Eve's cognitive challenges, I noticed that she was running out of steam by midafternoon, even though she napped daily. I presumed her weakened right side was slowing her down. Although she was faithfully practicing her hand-eye coordination exercises (bouncing balls, tossing balls hand to hand, standing on one foot for increasingly longer periods), she still walked crooked and looked to be on the verge of falling over when she was standing still. My intuition told me that her constant attention to correcting her balance was depleting her energy. I was exhausted just watching her.

If she could have afforded it, I would have ordered an hour physical therapy session every day. But she was stuck with that darned $5000 insurance deductible. Nevertheless, she still needed some sort of daily exercise. I, the clueless caregiver, would have to come up with a physical therapy routine matched to her capabilities.

This presented a problem. I knew zilch about physical therapy. Consequently, I'd be forced to estimate how much time she could exercise, where to draw the limits and when to push her. I was well aware that I could make a big mistake.

Whereas I didn't fear those parameters when it came to emotional/cognitive rehabilitation, I was timid and cautious about physical exercise. Of course, I discussed it with our friends, but nobody had a solution, until I mentioned it to a neighbor, a nurse who was into physical fitness.

"Why don't you check out the programs at the YMCA?" she suggested.

"Oh, that's way too expensive," I objected.

She countered, "They have reduced membership fees for hardship cases."

"Okay," I said, "but I don't think Eve can handle the class situation. She's so slow. I'd worry that she would be trampled on her way from the locker room to the gym."

"I'll bet they would allow you to accompany her," my friend retaliated.

At this point in the conversation, both of us realized I was arguing for my limitations. The truth was, when I saw that glimmer of hope, I became equally fearful of rejection. What if Eve didn't qualify for financial aid? Did I have a right to beg on her behalf? I paused a moment to consider the alternative: chubby, out-of-shape me leading exercise routines in the living room. I decided to respond more positively.

"Okay, I'll phone the membership director," I said. "It can't hurt to talk to her."

And so I set the YMCA meeting appointment, dragging Eve with me. Truly, I went into the meeting with very little hope that Eve would qualify for financial aid or that there was any class at Eve's ability level, or any instructor willing to take on the responsibility for Eve's safety, or that they would allow me to accompany Eve.

I was wrong on all four counts. The empathetic membership director listened patiently to my pleas. Before I had finished, she started the paperwork to enroll Eve in a low-impact water exercise class, taught by a certified therapy instructor. Plus, all fees were paid for by a scholarship fund. That's not all. Because I was the caregiver, I was also given a scholarship and enrolled in an aerobics class that gave me time to supervise Eve's shower and dressing needs. It was one more lesson I had to learn about not letting fear stand in the way of recovery—either Eve's or mine.

On the days when Eve didn't have class, I instituted a neighborhood walk routine for both of us. On those walks, I directed Eve to look up, down and sideways to stretch her growing ability to correct her balance in an ever-changing physical environment. As we walked and gawked, I'd quiz Eve about the flowers, birds and homes we encountered along the way.

By taking frequent walks with Eve, I became more confident in judging her limits and encouraging better performance. Within months, the results were more than amazing. I was skinnier! Eve actually began to push herself to do more. This was indeed a surprise because, overall, Eve was still minimally motivated to do most of her daily tasks.

I recall reading a stroke survivor's book in the early days of Eve's recovery, in the hope of getting a tip or two. Alas, what I got was a little jealous and a lot depressed. Unlike the author, Eve exhibited minimal motivation to do the grunt work she needed to do in order to get well. At first, I thought it was my perception problem. I couldn't perceive the flicker of the fire of desire in Eve to improve herself cognitively. Although I believed I had zeroed in on her primary lifelong motivations, I began to doubt my ability to motivate her. Perhaps my style of communication was too forceful, or not tough enough. Maybe I was too emotionally involved or, on the contrary, not caring enough. I varied approaches. I yelled at her and bargained with her. Sometimes I begged.

RECOVERING EMOTIONAL SENSITIVITY

Meanwhile Eve had a complaint of her own. At least two or three times a week, she'd pipe up, "I can't feel my emotions." Considering how much time I devoted to reading her nonverbal body language communication, I'm surprised how little importance I gave this verbalized self-assessment.

Oh, sure, we discussed it; but after ten minutes or so I'd dismiss it by saying, "Well, you never were very emotional. Remember in the beginning you couldn't physically feel hot or cold? And now you can. Maybe your emotions will come back in the same slow way." After a few months of listening to Eve's complaint, I finally acted on it. I arranged several sessions with a psychological counselor. They didn't go well. Eve was still having difficulty initiating conversations and her responses to questions were quick, short, not very thoughtful and sometimes just plain wrong. I had to be present. The few times I tried to let Eve do solo sessions, the therapist ended up requesting my presence after twenty minutes. Eventually, the therapist became frustrated, and so did I.

I tried another therapist, who suggested Eve write a short daily journal, recalling past important events and associated emotions. Then we spent the rest of the hour discussing my frustration with Eve's low-level motivation. By the end of the session, the therapist stated, "What we have here is an individual who has demonstrated above-average recovery despite below-average motivation."

"Is she just plain lazy?" I asked. The therapist shrugged.

When we returned home I pondered the question of laziness. Did it matter? I had vowed that my mission was solely to restore the old Eve, and not change her into some fictional character I wanted her to be. Yes, the Eve of old was lazy at times; but, truth be told, I considered myself lazier. And yet, I knew that if I was cognitively disabled, I'd be hitting the books for hours every day, trying to get my brain back. Other than our joint crossword-puzzle-solving routine, Eve wouldn't crack any of the problem-solving books I had bought her. She had accumulated a pile of them—brainteasers, mazes, logic problems, Mensa tests, creativity boosters. All were books that I was absolutely positive would have intrigued the old Eve. Yet she avoided them like the plague, much preferring to read cereal boxes, the small print on credit card bills, and phone books. (Oh, she liked reading novels and cozy mysteries; but I strictly enforced after-dinner-only leisure reading time.) Though I promised to rewrite her daily routine so she could work on her cognitive problem books all afternoon, she simply wouldn't do it.

After much thought, I arrived at my own evaluation of Eve's problem. As with everything I did with Eve, I stated the problem to myself in untechnical terms, so I would remain in touch with the reality of the situation. Eve lacked the emotional component of motivation. She had a limited emotional range and an inability to feel her emotions very well. I believed Eve had difficulty perceiving any problem, whether it was a housekeeping task or a mental exercise. By the time she perceived it, she was too tired to think of more than one solution. Often the first solution she thought of did not solve the problem. Consequently, her emotional responses were either disappointment at failure or boredom. As a result, Eve was more prone than ever to seek instant gratification—or nothing—versus working at a solution that gave her minimal emotional payback (which she could barely feel.).

Dutifully, I included the therapist's emotion-journaling exercise at the end of the day, before our crossword puzzle. I gave Eve a notebook for the assignment. A week later, I asked if I could see what she had written. She had described two events: her wedding (nervous) and her husband's death at a relatively young age (very sad). I involved myself in the process. Unfortunately, every session somehow involved memories of her husband, concluding with a discussion of how sad it was. This was not where I wanted Eve to direct her limited emotional energy. In the end, I was the one who was emotionally motivated to add more emotional spark to our lives.

For this I needed to focus the Eureka! strategy on activities specifically designed to encourage a positive (happy), emotional response.

Who in the world does this better than those masters of the one-minute motivational message, the creators of commercials and direct response advertising?

SUGGESTION:

In a relaxed state, pay attention to the routine activities in your lives. Perhaps Eureka! is already happening and you simply haven't recognized it yet. You'll find it in those activities that seem to motivate the patient to successful living. Make a note of them, even if you are not exactly certain why or what makes them a candidate for your emotional motivation purposes. Let it rest for a day and then see what intuition tells you tomorrow. Once you know what and why, you'll be able to maximize the Eureka! effect.

Trust the process.

19

How TV Advertisers Create Eureka!

It is time to start thinking about creating Eureka! on purpose. For that we can turn to the persuasion techniques the advertising professionals use to stimulate emotions, to inspire behavior changes and to encourage action.

You don't have to do anything yet—just read and *feel*. I am trusting that the simple action of reading about these advertising techniques will trigger memories, so you can feel how this aspect of Eureka! might trigger the patient's memories. Going one step further, I hope that this process helps you recognize opportunities you could use to create the over-the-top emotional Eureka! approach. Ultimately, I hope it inspires you to try to inspire the patient on that all-important emotional level. So now, let's see how the professionals create Eureka!

A long, long time ago, the college professor who taught my advertising communications class explained that the key to great advertising was to find the unique selling proposition of the product—and dramatize it.

He gave us an assignment. Pick any two breakfast cereals, toilet papers and airlines and compare the USPs (the unique selling propositions)—the product features that make them different. Five minutes into the assignment, anyone could see that the two featured in any category were more similar than different. But thanks to a clever copywriter, we understood that one airline was forever friendly while the other gave wings to its passengers; one toilet paper was soft while the other lasted longer; one cereal talked but the other was "G-r-r-reat!"

Thank goodness we caregivers don't have to sell look-alike products. All we have to do is come up with an activity or adventure that's unique, meaning different from the patient's everyday life. Then we figure out the unique selling proposition for the activity. We look for whatever makes it fun, exciting or enjoyable and we celebrate it with the patient. That's Eureka!

Think about all of the TV commercials you have watched in your lifetime. Granted, many are irritating. However, some are pure genius in the way they communicate their memorable, emotion-evoking, informational messages or calls-to-action. These commercials are the ones that make us giggle or ponder trick photography or fall in love with an irresistible celebrity spokesperson.

We caregivers can take a lesson from these powerful one-minute persuaders. Many contain helpful, creative brain rehabilitation techniques that we can borrow for the home-caregiving situation. These techniques can help us persuade the patient to control or show emotion, try exercising a frozen limb, limit an obsessive-compulsive behavior, bring back old familiar behaviors, become more social and retrieve those emotions that made the patient come alive in the past.

No doubt about it, the great commercials are caregiver textbooks on how to make a minute memorable. Remember the old-fashioned soup commercials that evoke feel-good memories from the past? You, too, can serve up an instant bowl of nostalgia. Others use high-impact emotional events to teach new lessons, such as trash bags falling apart to demonstrate the right way to take out the garbage. You, too, can teach those show and tell lessons. And how about the commercial that employs a visual or auditory technique that grabs attention and doesn't let go until it has delivered the message? You can hum a song and dance through a task to make it more enjoyable. There are more attention-attracting techniques including exaggerated situations, visual tricks and humor.

Last but not least there's my favorite emotion-triggering technique: anthropomorphization. It is not only the biggest word in this book; it's also one of the most powerful.

The dictionary defines anthropomorphization as the technique of endowing animals and inanimate objects with human qualities. I define it as an easy-to-master creative caregiver tool for making Eureka! moments memorable.

My favorite anthropomorphized "star" of commercial TV is the incorrigible but adorable duck who quacks the name of the insurance he sells. There are many other famous examples including the finicky cat, the grumpy candy, dancing raisins, talking dogs and oodles of animated cartoon characters. We listen to their persuasive sales pitches because they are so loveable. I'm sure you can think of more examples and, in fact, it's a good idea to make notes.

Here's one example of how I used anthropomorphization to inspire Eve. One fine spring day I decided that gardening would be a perfect rehabilitation task for Eve. It made sense. As long as I had known her, planting and nurturing a garden was Eve's pride and joy. So, on the occasion of our first nice spring day in our new home, I invested more money than I should have for flats of petunias, geraniums and three flowering potentilla shrubs for the front yard. We planted them together. It was fun and Eve appeared to be proud of her accomplishment. Afterward, I reminded Eve that she had agreed to trim, prune, weed and water her yard and garden for the season. Two weeks later, the flowers were drooping and the potentillas were dying of thirst. I couldn't believe what a dismal failure my idea was. I dragged Eve out into the yard.

"What happened?" I asked her. "Why don't you care about what you planted? These plants cost us a fortune."

"I do care," she said. "I guess I forgot." She shrugged. I was frustrated. Yelling did no good. The wasted money investment did not seem to faze her. The sad sight of drooping flowers and bushes didn't touch her soul, at least not enough for her to remember to take care of them.

To make matters worse, she still didn't seem to care very much, certainly not as much as I did. I pointed to the potentillas lined up along the driveway. "How could you do this to our little babies, Flopsy, Mopsy and Cottontail?" I wailed at Eve.

Just then, the potentillas cried out. "We want water. We're so thirsty. We want our mommy to give us a drink."

"Huh?" Eve was startled by the plaintive plea, emanating from me. (I'm a lousy ventriloquist; but who cares.)

The sobbing potentillas got her attention. I stoked the fire. I did not want to let go of the moment, so I talked fast and somewhat nonsensically. "Well you know, Eve, we adopted Flopsy, Mopsy and Cottontail when we took them away from the nursery. We took them away from their mommy. We promised the owner that we'd take good care of them. And now look at them. They are so forlorn, so sad. They need love. They were depending on you to be their mommy, and you don't seem to care."

"Please love us and take care of us, Mommy Eve," the potentillas begged in unison.

I knew I wasn't fooling Eve. She well understood the game I was playing. As I had hoped, Eve joined in the imaginary drama. (NOTE: I would never use this technique with someone who could not separate fact from fantasy.) But Eve really wanted to play the game, too.

"Oh, poor Flopsy, Mopsy and Cottontail. Don't cry. I'm sorry I neglected you little darlings," Eve said to the bushes. "I promise I'll never let you be thirsty again. I promise to weed and water you every day. Honest, I do."

Eve did—that summer and every summer thereafter. Six years later Flopsy, Mopsy and Cottontail Potentilla are alive and thriving. Eve proudly invites me to view their new baby blossoms every spring. She named the baby blossoms. We talk to them all summer long, encouraging them to grow. It's amazing how chatty potentillas are.

Was I being ridiculous? Truthfully, I have no shame when it comes to trying any technique I can think of to help my friend pick up the pieces of her mind and feel her emotions again. As with the quacking insurance duck or the finicky cat, the anthropomorphization technique never becomes old or boring. It helps me attract Eve's attention. She wants to be included in the drama. The technique helps her pay attention to the more mundane elements of life (as the duck does for "boring" supplemental insurance). Much of Eve's routine would be very boring indeed without an injection of humor, enthusiasm, creative exaggeration and over-the-top dramatization.

One more thought about anthropomorphization: Never underestimate the power of the real thing (meaning pets) to deliver meaningful messages to the patient. Above and beyond their ability to re-teach the patient to take responsibility for another creature's survival, pets can be a caregiver's best friend, in more ways than one.

I have worked in cahoots with our cats, Chuckles and Lola, to praise, admonish and offer various suggestions to Eve. For some reason, Eve pays more attention to what the cats tell her than anything I have to say. For instance, some days I can command Eve to pick up fuzzballs until I'm blue in the face. Far better to have Chuckles do the dirty work by saying, "Mommy, there are pieces of my fur all over the couch. It makes me sneeze." Eve never fails to pay attention to what Chuckles has to say.

Getting Eve to pay attention has always been a problem, even pre-aneurysm. Many years before her aneurysm, Eve consulted a therapist to help her deal with her husband's death and the onslaught of unfamiliar emotions she was feeling. During the sessions, the therapist would ask Eve to identify the emotion she was talking about. Generally, Eve couldn't do it. So the therapist gave her a list of all the emotions one could possibly feel. In telling this story to me, (pre-aneurysm), Eve laughed about how she'd always have to refer to the list in order to respond to the therapist's questions.

Maybe Eve's lack of attention to her feelings was amusing back then; but I wasn't laughing now. My entire subconscious approach to Eve's brain rehabilitation depended on my ability to get Eve to "pay attention" to her feelings, so that I could link today's emotion with yesterday's memories. Would my plan still work if she never has been able to feel her emotions very strongly?

I wondered and I thought about that. In her pre-aneurysm days, Eve resisted focusing on the moment. She was always easily distracted by the noise of everyday life. She would rather "keep moving" than pause to savor the emotion of the moment. Theoretically speaking, I was trying to link present day emotions with emotional memories she experienced before the age of seven, before her conscious, logical mind had developed. Most people can't consciously recall early childhood memories anyway. Whether Eve could recall them or not, these old memories still contained the most powerful emotional content Eve had ever experienced in her life. The part of the equation I could control was how much emotional impact I could bring to today's "memory."

It was my job to jolt those old memories with high-impact, emotion-triggering events in the "now." If I could then persuade Eve to focus on the present—to pay attention to the now—today's emotion would have more trigger power to bring back the "old" and to reinforce the "new." It was worth my efforts to wallop her subconscious with all the techniques and tricks I could use, primarily borrowed from the best of advertising. I had a minimal budget, so I would have to be very creative indeed.

My first project was to create motivational messages—like billboards—for the walls and mirrors of our home.

When we moved into our modest, "new" old home, I tried to make it look attractive in the traditional sense. I decorated the walls with paintings, photographs and plaques. But soon I realized that I needed to be far more practical and creative with that precious wall space. Unexpected guests would have to understand that our house was now officially designated as command headquarters for Eve's brain rehabilitation. I needed more room to display motivational messages, memory aids and creative emotion-retrieval helpers.

Every command center functions around an everchanging bulletin board and strategy chalkboard of one sort or another. For our purposes, I needed to invest in office supplies, to help "advertise" our Eureka! memory-making strategy.

First, I strategically positioned three bulletin boards in the utility room, Eve's bedroom and (sigh) the living room. For the kitchen and bath, I bought tape, thumbtacks and refrigerator magnets, plus two "erasable" boards for menu-making and grocery "inventory control." I bought a year's supply of sticky notes. My intention was obvious: any Eve-deed worth doing would be framed, highlighted, thumb-tacked, prominently plastered, or otherwise broadcasted on the wall where (hopefully) Eve would pay attention to it. Soon our house became a gigantic showcase for "brain" motivation billboards—the latest in home style brain rehabilitation décor.

As I learned back in my college days while studying the art and science of communications, billboards are the ultimate advertising vehicle. A great billboard combines a stunning visual—photograph or art—and a brilliant message in 10 words or less. With one picture and a few words, the billboard must capture attention and deliver a message. The really great billboards inspire desirable emotional response, teach an important fact and motivate action. With a little imagination, we can do the same.

In the home environment, creating emotional, motivational billboards is not as difficult as it might initially appear. For Eve, I simply selected her favorite landscape and vacation photos and taped a short motivational message on each. I also drew my own visuals. Of course, I wrote my messages billboard-style, because that's been my life work. However, the Internet, my web site and library books are filled with inspirational messages that the caregiver can select, print and paste.

I have also used old advertising slogans and popular song lyrics or titles to help Eve pay attention. She enjoys reading the motivational messages I dream up to reinforce the ad slogan or song title. Personally, I think she delights in watching my creative struggles. But this is good. It demonstrates to her that I believe bringing back her spirit is worth the effort. And it is.

SUGGESTION:

Some of you can jump right into this project. Select a favorite photo and a favorite slogan or words of wisdom— something that relates to how you want to motivate the patient. If you need a little help, you can start by posting a sticky note with a slogan, such as: Pay Attention or One Day at a Time on the photo. Or you can post the illustrated motivational messages from this book, after you or the patient colors them. I'll tell you about even more ways to creatively use this coloring project later in the book.

20

It's Showtime!
Maximizing the Eureka! Effect

As Eve proceeded through her daily routine, I realized our social calendar featured too few social activities. For Eve's sake and mine, this had to change.

Considering my limited time and energy, I could only do so much socializing on a regular basis, especially in later years when I was working a job.

However, intuition told me that if I could plan one activity a week with Eureka! potential, I could maximize the effect of the good emotional feelings and enthusiasm naturally generated by the activity. It would be like staging a theatrical production—starring the patient and featuring me (the caregiver) as director and supporting cast. Oh, I don't want to forget my other important role—the set designer. Actually, on the Eureka! stage, most of my time and energy is devoted to creating the scenario, so that I can sit back, relax, watch and wait for that Eureka! moment to happen as the adventure unfolds.

The way I figured, if I could guess when to expect that Eureka! moment, I could make better use of it for Eve's rehabilitation. I was confident I could read Eve's enthusiasm level by watching her eyes. So I focused on planning an adventure a week, designed to create eye sparkle. For at least two or three hours, I wanted my Eureka! activity to generate a holiday atmosphere filled with anticipation and excitement.

In other words, I wanted the Eureka! moment to be like the 4th of July, 2002, Eve's first major holiday celebration after the brain aneurysm.

That summer morning, the sun had risen out of the blue Lake Michigan waters into a clear, "forever" sky. The waves gently lapped the rocky ledge in the backyard of our shoreline home. Then, as now, we lived in Door County, a Midwest summer tourist destination. Eve's good friend, Cass, was driving up from Chicago. All week long Eve and I had cleaned and shined the house in happy anticipation of our visitor and the holiday festivities that were planned.

Our tiny town of Baileys Harbor traditionally celebrated the holiday with the cutest, hokiest parade down Main Street. The day was filled with sunbathing, singing songbirds and soaring seagulls, boat-watching, lemonade, homemade ice cream from the town's sweet shop, a walk along the shoreline, hamburgers on the grill, and the climax: fireworks over the water as viewed from our front-row seats in our own backyard.

I don't think Eve ever stopped smiling that day. But, more memorably, I remember the nonstop sparkle in her eyes. It lasted for several days, fanned by our frequent reminiscing sessions at break-fast, lunch and dinner. I don't know the technical terms to describe the improvements I saw in her mind/body/spirit, but I know Eve was a different person thereafter. She listened longer, nodded her head more, and responded more appropriately to situations in the home and when friends called on the phone, especially Cass.

Obviously, every day is not a holiday with visitors. I can't command a festive parade performance, nor can I arrange a fireworks display every night. However, there are some variables from that memorable occasion I can duplicate. One is to take advantage of the inherent beauty and variety of experiences offered by nature.

The other is to plan the day with activities that are unique and out of the ordinary for our lifestyle. They must be interesting to Eve and worth anticipating.

Most importantly, I've got to think up activities that inspire me to be enthusiastic and offer the opportunity for me to overdramatize or exaggerate the fun parts of the adventure. I don't need money or other people (although both are helpful) to create a unique Eureka! adventure for Eve and me. In planning the event, I need to consider not only my abilities and stamina, I have to evaluate Eve's energy level and estimate her ability to maintain her focus and pay attention to the now. We devote two to four hours for most of our weekly adventures.

Every Eureka! adventure is promoted to Eve à la the showing of coming attractions for a blockbuster movie. I tell Eve what we're going to do. Next, I tell her what we're doing while we're doing it. Finally, I tell her what we've done. In my telling, I always emphasize what I consider to be the climax of the day's adventure, the much anticipated moment of Eureka!

This is what makes the Eureka! adventure different from ho-hum, ordinary outings. It's more interesting, more challenging or more fun than Eve's everyday life. I extend the value of the adventure using the overdramatization concept and exaggeration technique borrowed from the advertising copywriter's approach to promoting a product. It's the idea of selling the sizzle instead of the steak.

Here's an example of a planned Eureka! adventure, a Sunday afternoon stroll several years ago.

Autumn was staging a grand finale in Door County when summer made a surprise appearance. I had scheduled that particular Sunday for my weekly adventure with Eve. The weatherman was predicting a storm for Monday. I had promised Eve we were going to see the fall colors before the wind blew away the leaves. Unfortunately, I had been too busy to write my weekly feature column for the local newspaper. It was due the next day. I didn't even have a topic for it. What to do?

"Aw, heck," I said to Eve, "I'm going to do what Scarlett O'Hara did in *Gone with the Wind*. I'll think about that tomorrow. Let's not waste this gorgeous day. How about if we take a walk to Sunset Park along the canal? You can wear your new top and pick out a cap." (Eve had a vast collection of sporty sun visors and baseball caps. We made selecting a cap a ritual part of any outdoor adventure.)

When we arrived at the park, this was the scene. Boats were cruising up and down the Sturgeon Bay Canal. Their sunlit sails seemed to glow against the red and copper colors of the maples lining the opposite shore. To our right, stormy purple clouds were gathering over Green Bay, contrasting sharply with the fluffy white puffs dotting a baby-blue sky on our left. And above, a flock of geese were descending, taking a break from their flight south to sunbathe on the beach. From out of the gaggle, one goose waddled toward us, honking a "hello". We chatted for a while, the goose and I. Eventually, Eve joined in. Meanwhile, a summerlike sun warmed our backs while the crisp Green Bay breeze reminded us that autumn would soon rule the day.

Of course, Eve saw what I saw, but not the way I saw it. I approached the moment like a kid set loose in a candy shop (or as an advertising copywriter selling a bowl of cereal). I searched out every unique or interesting attribute of the scene and communicated every detail to Eve, with over-the-top enthusiasm. If anyone was eavesdropping that day, I sounded like the play-by-play announcer on a radio broadcast of a football game.

Here's how I prepared for that moment on the spot. When we arrived on the scene, I took three deep breaths. I gave myself a suggestion to be enthusiastic. I added a prayer in case God was listening. I often ask God to help me help Eve to see, hear, taste and feel the activity as she would have pre-aneurysm. I can't make her do this; I can only hope for her. However, I can ask for help to be enthusiastic. Then I prove to myself this is all working by communicating aloud all the different reasons why I feel so enthusiastic.

Obviously, this requires me to pay attention to what is going on around me right now. Next, I tell Eve what my senses are seeing, touching, hearing, etc. and how it makes me feel. My hope, my goal, is to inspire an emotional reaction, however subtle, in Eve.

Here's how I sounded to Eve. "So, here we are on the Sturgeon Bay Canal on this beautiful day. Do you feel the sun on your back? Warm, isn't it? And yet the breeze off the water is cool. I can't believe it's October in Wisconsin. Are you comfortable? Look at the beautiful blue sky in the East. Uh-oh, do you see those clouds gathering in the West? That gray one looks like a witch on a broom. Bet it's going to storm tonight, don't you think? I love these Indian Summer colors, the burnt oranges and burgundies. Let's find a park bench where we can sit and relax near the beach. It'll be our front-row seat to watch boats on the canal.

"Look at the sails on that one. Here comes a motor boat, making big waves. Uh-oh. They look like they're going to collide. Whew. That was too close. Wonder how the people on the sailboat feel about that? Ahh, I'm getting sleepy. The sun is so warm. Hear that honking? It's a flock of geese somewhere. Where are they? Oh, here they come. They're going to land right on the beach in front of us. Boy, they're big. Look at those little ducks running away from them.

"Oh my, here comes a really big goose. Honk, honk, yourself. What did he say? Oh, he was just commenting about how crowded the beach is today. Now don't laugh, Eve. I swear that's what he said. Ask him yourself." (She does. He honks back. She says, "He wants to know if we brought a picnic lunch.")

"That reminds me, I'm getting hungry. How about you, Eve? Let's walk to town and get some nourishing ice cream. Two dips in a waffle cone? What flavors are you going to get? We'll celebrate summer's last hurrah. Wave goodbye to summer, Eve. We won't see it again for a long time."

And so it goes. Nothing I said sounded particularly brilliant. I asked a lot of questions, tossed out lots of feelings. I invited Eve's response all the time. Some questions were better than others at evoking emotional responses; but who cares? I believe that Eve realized on some level that I was trying for sensual, emotional reactions and in response, Eve rose to the occasion as best she could—physically, mentally and emotionally.

The enthusiasm I exhibit will always be contagious. No matter what Eve actually does or says, this will be a Eureka! activity. I am touching emotions that make memories and retrieving all similar emotional memories from the past. Go ahead; ask Eve if she remembers this ordinary day from several years ago. She'll tell you all about it—sights, sounds and feelings—from the day summer collided with autumn on the canal.

Most importantly, she'll tell her tale with a level of enthusiasm above and beyond anyone's expectations.

By the way, there was an extra added bonus to our field trip that day. When I returned home, the column virtually fell out of my head onto the writing pad. Eve offered to type it. Then she read my prose back to me, so we could both relive the memory. That's part of the Eureka! strategy, too. When you've created a great memory, keep feeding it.

SUGGESTION:

Let's have a dress rehearsal for creating your first purposeful Eureka! adventure. We'll do mine first, as an example.

Remember a few chapters ago when I told you my biggest regret was that I shoulda—coulda—woulda created a Eureka! day for my stroke-afflicted Dad. If I had read then what I just wrote now, here's what I would have done.

As I said, after the stroke Dad had become an emotionless couch potato. The highlight of his days was the Sunday afternoon telecast of Chicago Cubs baseball games. If I had been thinking, I could have made Sunday afternoon Eureka!

First I'd create the atmosphere by turning on a fan full-blast to simulate the always-blowing lake breeze that's so much a part of being at Wrigley Field, the Cubs' ballpark. Then we would turn off the sound on the TV. I would have recruited my brother to play the part of Cubs' announcer, Harry Carey, who saluted every home run with a joyful "Holy Cow!" and who led the fans in a boisterous rendition of "Take Me Out to the Ball Game" at the 7th inning stretch.

Meanwhile, I would have hawked beer and peanuts, punctuated with an occasional "Get your Red Hots here!" We would have kept score on "real" scorecards. I would ask Dad for the umpteenth millionth time what the shorthand symbol was for walking in a run or flying out to center. We would have "cheered and booed and raised a hullabaloo" for the sake of seeing that sparkle in Dad's eyes.

Your turn to dress-rehearse. For now, just think about what might make a great adventure for you and your loved one. In the next chapter, I'll give you more tips on how to make Eureka! happen and how to maximize its effect.

21

Do It Yourself Eureka! Adventures

Since our budget was limited, choosing our Eureka! activities presented a weekly challenge. Obvious activities such as concerts, plays, fancy dining and weekend trips were not feasible. These were all things Eve and I previously enjoyed. But the medical bills and diminished savings put an end to all that.

What did we lose? Well, all of the aforementioned have inherent drama. There's an exciting climax contained in each of them: the final act of the play, the favorite song at a concert, the dessert at the dinner, and the adventure of a trip. These organized activities take the pressure off the caregiver to invent and create the Eureka! moment.

On the other hand, the more professionally staged activities one can afford, the harder the caregiver has to work to make them outstanding Eureka! moments. For the wealthy, dining out isn't a treat; it's routine. For those with friends galore, or a country-club lifestyle, a party invitation isn't an extraordinary event. This diminishes the Eureka! effect. (Ho-hum, we've been invited to another gala ball.) Part of the Eureka! strategy is that the event is out-of-the-ordinary.

Therefore, I've come to the gratifying conclusion that Eureka! caregivers on a budget have a definite advantage. Once the caregiver learns the simple Eureka! memory-making strategy, all sorts of interesting, stimulating, fun and low cost entertainment ideas become candidates for the weekly Eureka! adventure. (Note: These activity suggestions are not replacements or alternatives to professional rehabilitation therapy or medical care. I checked out my Eureka! strategy for Eve with physicians, nurses and therapists. I suggest you do the same.)

Over the years, Eve and I have visited innumerable parks and gardens, trekked wildflower trails, strolled dozens of beaches and oohed and aahed as the sun set over the bay. We participated in free festivals, viewed parades, listened to open-air concerts, people-watched at parks and window-shopped in town. Our major expenses were occasional ice cream cones or coffee-to-go.

However, I did invest my time in planning the activity. In preparation for any particular outing, I'd present an invitation to Eve, outlining the plan for the activity. "Hey, Eve, do you want to join me while I take photographs of dandelion fields and cherry blossoms tomorrow? If it's sunny, we can go for a drive on the country roads. See the cows. Watch the corn grow. You can help me look for golden farm fields. We can also visit some farm markets. While I'm photographing their cherry orchards, you can see if they have a good price on cherry pie. It will be our treat for the weekend. You can shop for it while I photograph; or you can help me find good shots out in the field. Does that sound like fun, Eve?"

Here's Eve's typical response: "Ooh. Good. Something different. It beats doing laundry." Eve always tries to be cool; but I can tell when she's excited. I look for the sparkle in her eyes.

I am guessing that the Eureka! climax for this particular activity—the Unique Selling Proposition—will be Eve's purchase of cherry pie. Eve does have a sweet tooth. Then too, the sight of spring scenery after an interminably long Wisconsin winter might bring Eve a feeling of joy. I know I'm anticipating the country ride, so I won't have to work at generating enthusiasm.

"Okay, Eve, if tomorrow is a nice day, be ready to take off at 2:00 for our adventure. I need those afternoon shadows for photography." (Heaven forbid that I get up early to see the morning shadows.)

I've set the stage for Eve to expect an adventure in nature and I've promised cherry pie. I've asked her to help me in my artistic pursuit to photograph the countryside. I have my motivation. Hers is to purchase the dessert treat for our weekend meals. I've prepared her for some stimulating social interaction at the always-friendly farm market. With such a good plan, I can relax and leave myself "open" to recognize any unexpected Eureka! fun we encounter along the way.

I don't assume she realizes all the motivations, so I bring them up in conversations and reinforce them frequently throughout the preparation time.

By the time I'm ready to depart on my photo mission, Eve is dressed and ready to go. She surprises me by remembering to bring two bottles of water. I compliment her on her thoughtfulness, her looks and her promptness. (I always point out her cognitive and emotional successes as I see them.)

Before we leave, I ask if she's checked the house. This responsibility reinforces the importance of personal safety for her and her responsibility to ensure my safety, too. I tell her frequently that she's in charge of the house. After several of these ventures, she has gotten the message that she doesn't leave the premises without checking the cats' whereabouts, their food and water supply, that all appliances are turned off and a night light is turned on. (Locking doors is impolite where we live.)

Eve has also double-checked her wallet to make sure she has plenty of money for the pie. Interestingly, Eve always feels better if she's in charge of the money. Either she is remembering that I habitually forget it or she wants to be in control. Since managing money is an important survival tool, I generally hand over the money management to her whenever we go to the store or out to a restaurant. I have also emphasized that credit card usage is reserved for emergencies. Nothing is paid with credit without discussing it first. Initially, I instituted this to counter her compulsive tendencies after the brain aneurysm. Now, considering the new economic situation, it's an absolute rule in our household. I sure am glad I trained myself to practice what I preach.

Finally, we're off. As I drive out of town, I give Eve the assignment of finding a cherry orchard with pastures overflowing with sunny dandelions. I'm looking for dramatic color contrast, I tell her. Now Eve has a creative, artistic "mission" and I have a helper as we begin our Eureka! adventure.

"Look over there!" she shouts. "What a great picture! Pull off the road. We'll walk back and I'll show you the picture."

And so I do. We walk back. I'm quiet; this is Eve's show. "Stop," Eve commands as she frames a photo with her hands. "Look, there are the cherry blossoms. See the dandelions between the trees. Oh look, if you take the picture from here, you can include that old red barn." Eve's eyes are sparkling. She's excited. And most importantly, she's created the first Eureka! memory of the day, ten minutes into the adventure. I snap several pictures, including one featuring smiling Eve.

The rest of the adventure proceeds somewhat according to my hoped-for plan. Eve chats with a farm market owner and purchases her cherry pie. ("It's frozen," Eve apologizes to me. "They used last season's cherries for the filling. But I promise it'll taste fresh after I bake it.") Before we leave, I buy two cherry caramels for the ride home, for immediate gratification.

We also review the day as we drive. Not wanting to waste a great adventure, we review the day again on the weekend, while we are enjoying the pie. I always ask Eve first to lead us down Eureka! memory lane. If she forgets, I can embellish her account with the details I (miraculously) remember. If it's a photo field-trip, we review all the photos on the computer, too. Thanks to the magic of digital photo workshop programs, we can lighten, darken, crop and even change colors and effects. It makes us feel very creative. Plus, it doesn't cost a penny.

From our experience of dozens of Eureka! adventures, I've learned that they work best when Eve has at least a day to prepare herself. They are more memorable if I can include social interaction in the adventure. The outing is also more memorable if we treat ourselves to something tasty. The adventure should have an obvious beginning and an end, with a climax in-between. The activity is limited to the amount of time Eve is able to "pay attention", generally no more than three hours.

In addition, I've learned to review the day, on our way back home or, at the latest, that evening. Otherwise, she'll forget. I review the memory again later in the week, adding more information or triggering the senses by using photos of the day, food or some funny, interesting, emotion-related anecdote. (i.e. "I saw John Doe again while Chuckles and I were at the vet. He's the owner of the farm market. His dachshund had a sore paw. Poor little thing.")

But by far the most important element in any adventure is my level of enthusiasm for the outing. Most often, that's what creates the emotional impact that makes the day memorable and the activity Eureka! I am positive that my enthusiasm is contagious.

TREASURE HUNTS

Here's another easy Eureka! activity idea you can customize to please yourself and the patient. Shopping offers the caregiver an additional opportunity to create another weekly adventure. And why go on an ordinary shopping trip when you can go Eureka! "treasure hunting" together?

In recent years, Eve has demonstrated that she is capable of handling regular grocery shopping and a trip to Walmart for household essentials. However, we live in a farming area that is rich in wonderful specialty stores that include a local cheesemaker; a butcher shop that offers farm-fresh pork; a homemade maple syrup processor; a fresh lake perch purveyor; farm markets with apples, cherries and veggies; a jams and jellies merchant; and a homemade pickle-packer. If we are going to purchase these items anyway, it's well worth the drive and a few pennies more to get the best taste available, especially if I can engage Eve in a Eureka! memory session in the process. I can turn ordinary dinners into Eureka! by helping Eve recall how much fun we had buying the homemade hot dog relish, the farm-fresh corn or the world's best white cheddar cheese.

But you don't need a specialty store to create Eureka! We can do the same with a bimonthly trip to our very favorite drugstore, Walgreens. What's so special about this drugstore chain? If you asked Eve that question pre-aneurysm, she would have said, "It's just a drugstore." But if you asked me, a person who has often been strapped for cash, I would tell you Walgreens is the best source for fun gift ideas on a budget, great unexpected deals on essentials and lots of shopper surprises throughout the store. It's always been a treasure hunt waiting to happen for me. You just need the right attitude going in the door. (Eve is beginning to understand this because I always treat her to a fresh, new crossword puzzle book from the fun-to-peruse magazine rack.)

Every town has a store like this, usually a drugstore. When Eve and I lived near Sedona, Arizona, albeit one of the wealthier towns in the West, we found a Rite Aid drugstore along the main drag that featured bargains galore. We loved that shopping experience. As I recall, we found several unique Noah's Ark replicas to add to Eve's collection – all priced under $10. Plus, they had the cutest, cheapest, red rock T-shirts in town and a vast selection of tiny toiletries that delighted our house guests from Chicago.

Even in the heart of a tourist area like our Door County, Wisconsin, a fascinating shopping experience awaits everyone (including macho guys) at Nelson's True Value Hardware in Baileys Harbor. Nelson's was always a must-see stop on our family vacation agenda over fifty years ago. It hasn't changed one iota. The main floor is packed with eclectic merchandise, some of it decades old and priced accordingly. Where else could I buy 5-year-old picture calendars for a buck? But the real find is on the basement level, where bin upon bin features every screw, nut, nail and widget known to man. You can still buy onesies and twosies and replacement parts for vintage appliances. It's a riot.

These are the types of stores where you can set up your Eureka! adventure as a quest to solve a household problem, enjoy a treasure hunt to find your item, solve your problem on a budget and come home with another Eureka! memory notch in your belt. It all depends on your enthusiastic attitude and your willingness to search out adventures.

PLAY DAY AT HOME

Hopefully, I've underwhelmed you with how easy it is to create do-it-yourself Eureka! adventures away from home. However, I haven't forgotten how challenging it was just to leave the house and go anywhere with Eve in early recovery. Back in those first months, buckling Eve's seat belt for a car ride was an ordeal. She couldn't comprehend the concept of safety or belt buckling, and her frozen shoulder prevented her from doing it by herself. I needed to pack a diaper bag and a change of clothes, just in case. A quick bathroom stop on the road wasn't so simple from my point of view. (Those stalls aren't built for two.)

In addition, Eve was unaware of her bodily needs and functions. I felt it was my duty to not embarrass her in public, even though she could not feel that emotion. I had to consider the chance I might have to wipe her nose, or cut up her dinner at a restaurant, if she couldn't or wouldn't pay attention to what was happening.

In those early days, I was a "beginner" at purposefully creating Eureka! memory-making adventures. Had I known what I was doing back then, I woulda—coulda—shoulda come up with more ideas. If you're in a similar situation, here are examples of early "adventures" for creating Eureka! memories at home.

From the beginning, every therapist in the world suggested family photo scrapbook reviews as a great memory recall exercise. On the surface, the suggestion seemed logical; but it didn't work for us. First, I had only known Eve for ten years. Her scrapbooks contained oodles of photos of people I did not know. I couldn't prompt her to recall faces or occasions which meant nothing to me. Even her wedding pictures were useless for my purposes. Secondly, all of those photos minimally captured Eve's attention. Even stunning photos of the European countryside from Eve's college year in Rome did little to spark her interest. Without a clue as to most of the stories behind the photos, I simply couldn't help Eve relate to her foggy memories.

I also discovered that photos from our shared vacations, or from the years we lived in Sedona's Red Rock Country, did little at face value to generate any enthusiasm on Eve's part. That is, until the snowy Sunday afternoon we transformed a ho-hum photo review into a vicarious vacation experience for Eve and me.

We were sitting at the kitchen table, watching the umpteenth blizzard of the season inundate us with more snow, when I heard myself wistfully say, "This would be a whole lot easier to take if we were planning a trip to Cancun next week." Eve smiled and nodded, and a light bulb blinked in my brain.

"Of course we can go on a trip, Eve. We can leave this afternoon. Just give me an hour to make the arrangements." Eve smiled again. Was that curiosity, anticipation, or doubt twinkling in her eyes?

"We'll put you in front of the TV for a little bit, Eve. You watch some golf while I run down to the convenience store for trip supplies," I said as I pulled on my boots. Even I was getting a little excited now.

I raced down to the convenience store and paid too much money for corn chips, salsa and fizzy lime water. Back home, I searched out our Cancun vacation photos and a sombrero-style straw hat for me and Eve's beloved Cancun souvenir sun visor for her. I draped a serape over the table, set out the chips, dip and water, and put a marimba band CD on the player. I danced over to the dining table.

"Ole, Eve. Let's cha-cha down memory lane with our photos. Look at those bright red parrots. Remember the parrot preserve at

Xcaret Park? That one was eating chips out of your hand. And here's the butterfly meditation grove. Ooh, I think we've got some plastic butterfly souvenirs in the dresser drawer. Let me get them. We'll hang one from the lamp – and the other from my ear. Ha. Ha. We'll pretend we're back there at the Mayan village, looking out over the gulf and the Caribbean. Feel that ocean spray?" The more I talked, the more I remembered; story after story, gleaned from that week's vacation. Eve even remembered a couple of memories I forgot, like watching the live rodeo while munching a lunch of tortillas at Xcaret Park and snorkeling down the underground river.

Oh, yes, we had a wonderful tropical vacation that snowy afternoon. (Wish you were here!) What I lacked in money, I made up for with a wealth of memories that had Eureka! potential for my storytelling.

And what did that afternoon do for Eve cognitively or emotionally? It snapped her out of the winter doldrums; it evoked an emotional response; it focused her attention. It carried her through to dinner, and perhaps inspired her insistence that she could and would set the table properly and try her hand at taco-making later in the week.

For me, the caregiver, the afternoon offered a much-needed break from that "powerless" feeling of not having a clue as to how to reach Eve. I did reach her. And that gave me hope that I could do it again and again.

Here's another patient/caregiver activity that is as powerful as it is simple. Coloring pictures with crayons is such an easy way to create Eureka! at home. This activity triggers those essential emotional memories formed before age seven, when the developing conscious mind starts editing memory content and watering down the emotional impact of memories of good times and good feelings.

Coloring is emotionally stimulating, yet relaxing. It forces the patient to pay attention to the present for a brief period. It is immediately gratifying and almost every picture is a setup for success. Honestly, who could argue that coloring cows bright yellow in a field of pink under a chartreuse sky isn't creative? Right?

In addition, when the caregiver participates in the process—by coloring his/her own picture—both patient and caregiver reap rewards of a shared artistic experience. The door is open to both participants' subconscious minds. The creative energy flow and communication takes place at the intuitive level. Meanwhile, conscious communications are enhanced. Both caregiver and patient are better able to pay attention to the moment in the relaxed state of mind that coloring pictures creates.

I've discovered that when Eve and I are sharing a creative experience, it is the optimal time to deliver important communications to her. It is easier to motivate her. In fact, any type of "message" carries more emotional impact (and is therefore more memorable) during the creative coloring process.

That's why the last chapter of the book offers coloring pages. Both caregiver and patient can reap the benefits of thoughts and feelings evoked by the motivational meditations that accompany the pictures. As I mentioned in the advertising techniques chapter, the best billboard ads seek to create a relaxed, welcoming environment for delivering their dramatized or exaggerated messages. Unfortunately for them, advertisers also have to clamor for the audience's attention in a noisy, busy and indifferent environment. When you and the patient are quietly coloring together, you've already automatically created the ideal environment to coax, persuade and suggest changing behaviors and attitudes to help the patient function, cope and feel emotions.

By the way, even a paralyzed patient can participate by selecting crayon colors for the caregiver to use. You've noticed, I'm sure, that simply watching someone else color can be an all-involving experience. It's not optimal; but it is engaging.

Here's all the "equipment" you need for do-it-yourself Eureka!, indoors or outdoors.

First, you need ideas for an activity. For example: a picnic in the park; a trip to the zoo; a wildflower walk; an escape to the beach; treasure hunting; window-shopping; or an afternoon at a not-too-crowded mall; a drive along country roads; a visit to your old stomping grounds; homemade lemonade on the deck; a Frisbee toss in the backyard; bird watching out your window; making a big deal out of a televised sports event; or watching an all-time favorite movie with popcorn (and much more real butter than you'd ever get at the theater). Parties with family and friends are great. (They were rare occasions for us.) The most important thing to remember is that the patient should be the center of attention much of the time. Better yet, the guests could be advised in advance that bringing a souvenir and a memory of a shared experience with the patient would be most helpful for creating that emotional, social Eureka! adventure.

Second, you need to enthusiastically communicate your plan to the patient at least several hours before it happens (a day before is best). That way, you can build anticipation. Ignore any bah-humbug or so-what reactions from the patient. Keep on trucking with your enthusiastic approach. As you "talk up" the activity, concentrate on what you think (or, better yet, intuitively feel) will be the unique selling proposition—the Eureka! moment that makes it memorable.

Third, you need to practice relaxation so your stress level is under control. A relaxed approach helps you pay attention to the moment. It also frees you to watch for any Eureka! moments that might pop up, so you can maximize their effect.

Fourth, is simply to do it. Add color commentary or play-by-play descriptions as you go along. Pay attention and look for contrasts, coincidences, surprises and emotion-evoking happenings.

Fifth, be sure to review all the fun you had making the Eureka! memory out of whatever activity. Digital photo reviews on the computer can indelibly impress the subconscious mind and enhance recall.

Sixth, pay attention to the patient's behavior over the next few days. See if you can attribute any positive progress directly to the Eureka! activity. If so, plan to do it again and again.

SUGGESTION:

Here are two checklists to help you start planning Eureka! adventures for two. One is for outdoor Eureka! adventures; the other is for indoor Eureka! adventures. You'll find the indoor coloring project, with more suggestions for transforming it into a Eureka! adventure, at the end of Chapter 23.

EUREKA! OUTDOOR ADVENTURES CHECKLIST

❑ Set a day and a time limit in consideration of patient's energy level.

❑ Choose an out-of-the-ordinary activity (perhaps a nature walk, art fest, beach or mountain day trip).

❑ Check your enthusiasm level every step of the way. If it's waning, "act as if".

❑ Tell the patient the plan. (Focus on the Unique Selling Proposition of the Eureka! memory you want from the trip).

❑ Do it! (During the trip tell your patient what you see/hear/touch/taste/smell, or whatever is interesting, emotional or unique.)

❑ Give the patient a task to "accomplish" on the trip. (Compliment or reward the patient, as appropriate.)

❑ Take photos, if possible.

❑ Treat yourselves to candy, ice cream, coffee, any mouthwatering treat.

❑ Review the trip on the way home or later that evening. Encourage the patient to express the day's events in his or her own words. You can embellish the details.

❑ Review the trip again several days later, using the photos, any leftovers from the taste-treat or other souvenirs. Once again, encourage the patient to tell the story. Your role is to embellish details and emphasize the emotions experienced.

EUREKA! INDOOR ADVENTURES CHECKLIST

❑ Choose a date and time in consideration of the patient's energy level.

❑ Pick an activity. Choices may include family get-togethers, jigsaw puzzle sessions, TV movies or sports specials, coloring projects, etc.).

❑ Check your enthusiasm level at every step, remembering to "act as if" when it is waning.

❑ Announce the activity to the patient ahead of time, focusing on its unique or emotional aspects.

❑ Select props to enhance the emotional impact. This may include party decorations, hats, music, food.

❑ If it is a group adventure, invite supportive people who will add to the emotional impact (because you'll be asking them for help).

❑ If it's just the two of you, do something different, such as dressing up, that signals that this is a special event to the patient. Don't forget to invite your pets.

❑ Do the activity. Keep the chatter going, focusing on emotions and anything unique or humorous.

❑ Go over the top with compliments or rewards for the patient.

❑ Review the experience later that day, focusing on those emotional Eureka! moments, memories and taste-treats.

22

Eureka! And Éclairs!! Rewards for the Patient and the Caregiver

One ordinary winter's day, I received an extraordinary phone call at work from the local YMCA membership director. It was the same woman who had granted Eve the all-expense paid membership three years before and every year thereafter.

She said, "I have two favors to ask of you. First, could you please feature our annual fundraising drive in your weekly column?"

That was easy. "Yes," I happily agreed. As the winter progressed, I was running out of topics to write about in our now deserted Door County tourist area.

"Thanks. Secondly, I'd like to know if it's okay with you, as Eve's caregiver, if I call and ask her to be one of the keynote speakers for our fundraising kickoff. She'll have to give a short speech at the event to our directors, volunteers and major supporters."

I caught my phone before it fell on the floor. I stammered into the receiver. "Well, sure, I guess. Um, has Eve been talking up a storm at the 'Y' when I'm not around?"

A memory of our first and last three-way meeting flashed through my mind. That was the day I enrolled Eve in the "Y" program. I vaguely recalled having to kick Eve in the shins (gently, of course) in order to get her to respond to the membership director's questions. Had things changed that much since then?

"She's doing very well in her water-exercise class," the membership director said. "We want her to talk about what the scholarship means to her."

"Wow. It's okay with me," I said. "Just give me ten minutes before you call her at home. Let me call her first."

And so I did. Eve was thrilled; I told her that she'd have to think up her own speech, if she wanted to accept the invitation. Eve seemed to understand and she was willing. I was the one who was nervous. As often as I endeavored over the years to set up Eve for success, I worked equally as hard to avoid opportunities for public failure. I was always alert to the possible need of removing Eve from a social situation before she got too tired to make sense, or she was unable to correctly respond to social cues. I felt it was part of my caregiving duty to not embarrass her publicly, whether she was aware of it or not.

Talk about motivation, though; this invitation could be a biggie—the mother of all Eureka! memory-making adventures. Eve wanted to give the speech and my greatest personal challenge was to let her go and do it.

When I came home from work that evening, we chatted about Eve's speech. I asked her to tell me in a sentence or two how she understood the topic for her speech. Happily, Eve nailed it. Then I told her she had two weeks to write it. I wanted to listen to her rehearse it, but only once. I promised her and myself that I would not rewrite the speech. Then I asked her if that made sense and if she was okay with it. From that moment on, I relinquished control. (Boy, that was much harder than I thought it would be.)

On the night of the fundraiser kickoff, Eve looked stunning, dressed in her snazzy black blazer, setting off her silver hair. Her eyes sparkled with anticipation. Usually she's tired by 7:00; but not that night. Eve had energy, and an aura of excitement surrounded her.

The "Y" was the place to be in Door County that night. Before the ceremony began, Eve and I sampled the "everything chocolate" buffet. I nervously picked at a cream-filled candy or two. Eve was wolfing down brownie bites, followed by chocolate cherry chasers. She licked her fingers gleefully.

"Why don't you save some calories to celebrate after you've given your speech?" I suggested.

"I plan to." Eve winked at me and pointed at a nearby table. "I'm saving the éclairs over there for dessert." My, she was in a good mood. If I were giving a speech in ten minutes to a room filled with a couple of hundred people, I'd be a nervous wreck. As a matter of fact, I was.

We were seated at a banquet table at the back of the room. The membership director walked over and sat down at the table. "Are you nervous?" she asked Eve.

"Nope," Eve replied as she continued chomping on chocolate.

The membership director looked at me and raised an eyebrow. I shrugged and stuffed a white frosted chocolate pretzel in my mouth. I have never liked them.

I spoke. "Now, Eve, remember that if you forget your speech you can always read it." I pointed at the white note-filled index cards next to her plate. I relaxed a little. If all else fails, I thought, I know Eve is a good reader.

Eve nodded as the YMCA program director tapped the microphone on stage, signaling the beginning of the program. Thankfully, Eve stopped chomping. The membership director touched Eve's shoulder and pointed to the staging area for the speakers. "You'll be on in about 15 minutes," she whispered to Eve, as she flashed her watch. "I'll let you know when it's time."

Then the moment arrived. Eve gracefully rose from our table and successfully navigated around and through the maze of dessert tables to the other side of the huge room.

"She's up next," the membership director whispered to me. I nodded and, as I did, I caught a glimpse of something white peeking out from under Eve's dessert plate. Yep, it was the note cards for her speech.

I gulped and grabbed the cards. My first thought was to run

them over to Eve. My second thought was to let go and let God take care of Eve. Anyway, it was too late. Just then the emcee introduced her. Eve was on her way to the stage.

"Oh my God," I muttered to the membership director, as I fanned my face with the cards. She rolled her eyes up toward heaven. There was only time for a quick prayer, as the director adjusted the microphone to accommodate little Eve's height.

Eve began to speak. I took a deep breath to relax, and sat back in my chair. I was floored. Eve's speech was crisp, rhythmic and—most surprising of all—emotional and motivational. For nearly ten minutes, Eve entertained the audience with her description of how she was when she came in to the "Y" and how she had progressed slowly but surely, regaining her physical strength, balance and endurance along the way.

She made the point about how her financial situation required her to ask for assistance. She told her story with dignity. Then she dramatically paused and wowed the audience with a smile. With a loud and clear emotional plea, Eve asked the audience to write a check to help others recover from their disabilities and to exercise to build their strength. The audience applauded. Eve bowed. I wiped the tears from my eyes. The membership director smiled. Judging from the surprised look on their faces, a few veteran staff members in the audience realized the miracle they had just witnessed.

The program ended. Eve returned to the table. We put on our winter coats. I nudged her toward the dessert table. We wrapped up two éclairs "to-go" in a napkin and headed home. We had proven to ourselves that "We will get better together". We retired to the kitchen table to enjoy our just desserts.

Eve placed the éclairs on a festive plate, as I realized that the night's events had demonstrated again that the Eureka! strategy works. My mission as Eve's caregiver was to provide an emotionally stimulating scenario that had the potential to motivate Eve. But the process demanded that I relinquish the need to control the outcome. Once I relaxed and stepped aside, Eve's creative brain could rise to the occasion and heal itself.

Eureka! I did what a good brain caregiver is supposed to do. I grabbed the biggest éclair and took a bite before Eve could stop me.

23

Color Your Way to Eureka!
A 21-Day Motivational Strategy

Right about now, you deserve a vacation. It's a nice thought, if you have the time to take one. Perhaps when the patient gets better, you'll find a way.

This of course presumes you'll be healthy enough to accompany the patient. Are you taking care of yourself? That's the question I've been asking you throughout this book. If not, now is the time to start. Never, ever underestimate the power of stress to debilitate the caregiver emotionally, mentally and most especially, physically. From aching muscles, depression, anxiety to a host of other illnesses, prolonged stress has been known to bring down the best of us.

You want to be around to take that celebratory vacation with the patient, don't you? Then how about taking 60 minutes today to practice being stress-free and relaxed, just like you would on a real vacation.

It's easy, if you are willing to try. I can guarantee this plan will not work unless you "con" yourself into trying it—one day at a time for 21 days. I've made it so very simple, even I follow it. Incidentally, 21 days is the accepted period of time needed for repeating a daily action until it becomes a habit.

Whether or not you practice the program I've laid out here,

you'll still be devoting at least an hour a day to controlling stress and trying to motivate yourself. Trust me on this. It's all too easy to get swallowed up by the everyday challenges of brain caregiving. Saving "me" has never been quite this challenging, or as necessary, as it has been the past eight years of caregiving. If you can't survive and thrive, how will you help the patient do it?

Here's how the plan works. For the next 21 days, you'll be setting aside one hour (divided into practical segments) for your emotional and mental health. Don't feel guilty. As you'll see, you can actually share part of this hour with the patient.

Each day begins with the reading of a motivational meditation, which can be found at the end of this chapter. While you contemplate how the day's message might work in your life, you'll begin coloring a picture. Don't laugh. Just ask any therapist. Coloring pictures is a soothing, stress-relieving therapy that's easy, inexpensive and fun. It allows you to quickly bypass logical left-brain constraints and enter the creative realm where you can make intuitive, inspired connections.

If your patient is capable, he can color with you (or watch as you color) and both of you can discuss or contemplate the message. Limit yourself to 15 minutes of coloring in the morning. In the early evening, while you finish coloring the picture, take another 15 minutes to review the meditation to see how it worked for you during the day. This is what makes these meditations "different". You are holding yourself accountable for practicing positive behavior during the day. If possible, you can both discuss your achievements while coloring. Hopefully you'll have encountered a little miracle during the day to place on your gratitude-with-a-twist list later on.

The final half-hour is your personal intense relaxation time devoted to preparing you for a good night's sleep. It's worth the time when you consider that sleeping takes up a third of the day. It doesn't take much effort to increase the quality of those sleep hours. As we have previously discussed, warm bubble baths, hot showers, soothing tea, melatonin-rich cherry juice, a thoughtful daily gratitude list and a progressive relaxation countdown to dreamland can all become part of your private daily relaxation routine.

After a few days of doing this, you'll be asking me: "Who needs a vacation to relax?" Not only will your days and nights feel more relaxing; you'll actually be creating the home environment where Eureka! can happen to both of you. Little annoyances will disappear, stress will be alleviated, and eventually you'll see that you are handling challenges and crises more effectively and creatively. Each day will become an interesting adventure for you and the patient.

5 TOOLS FOR CREATING THE EUREKA! ENVIRONMENT

Following are five handy-dandy tools to help make relaxation your reality. These emotion-stabilizer tools will help you manage the stresses that pop up in everyday life. Using them regularly will also help you deal with crises more effectively. You have my word that at least one caregiver in this world has managed to use these tools and caregive at the same time.

AMAZING STRESS-O-METER

Every doctor wears a stethoscope. Every nurse carries a thermometer. And every caregiver can proudly display his/her own brand-new, custom-colored Stress-O-Meter.

Seriously, this is the best stress control product on the market. It's easy to use. It's economical, too. It incorporates the same principles as expensive biofeedback training, yet costs you nothing but a little time and effort. Your Stress-O-Meter is free. All you need to do is snip it out of the book or photocopy it. It's also on my Web site (Eurekamaster.com) if you want to print out a larger version. Then color it. By the time you're finished, you will have taken the first step to automatically and intuitively knowing how to gauge your stress level at any given time during the day. Armed with that information, you can use the simple relaxation methods—such as three deep breaths —to lower the stress level.

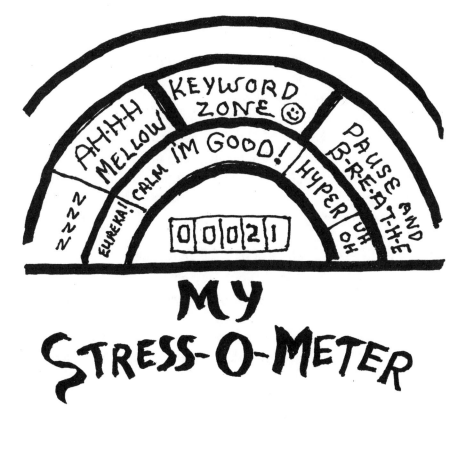

MY STRESS-O-METER

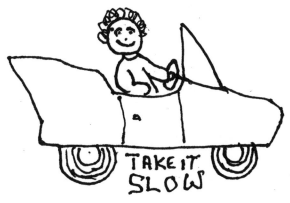

TAKE IT SLOW

So, before you begin your 21-day program, take ten minutes to color your Stress-O-Meter. First, color the calm zone with your favorite color. Next, color the stress areas a shocking shade of red, orange or fuchsia. While you are coloring the meter, imagine how all those stress levels feel.

When you feel stressed, take three deep breaths and concentrate on bringing down your stress level from the "Danger" zone to the "Calm/I'm Good" zone. "Mellow" is generally reserved for late evening. Carry the Stress-O-Meter in your purse, pocket or wallet and refer to it often – until you have it memorized. Keep practicing until you get it. Practice using it for 21 days before you "judge" whether it's helping.

YOUR PERSONAL MOTIVATING AD SLOGAN

"Do it." "Try, try again." "Never say never." "Easy does it."

Yes. You, too, can now be the proud owner of your very own stress-reducing, relaxation-motivating ad slogan. Take a few minutes now to think of a favorite phrase you can silently recite (in your head) to accompany your three deep breaths and relaxation routines. Examples might include: "slow down"; "peace"; "calm"; "I am serene" and "now is the time" (that's mine—you can use it, too). Or you can use a song title or an ad slogan. Practice saying your personal ad slogan while taking a deep breath during the 21 days—and beyond—until it becomes automatic. The more you practice using your personal ad slogan while breathing deeply, the more powerful both relaxation tools become. By the way, you can always change your mind. If you think of a new slogan for yourself, use it. Note: Do not obsess about the words. You'll soon realize that it's the emotion that counts.

MAGIC PROBLEM-SOLVING BOX

Somewhere in your house you have a shoebox, jewelry case, cigar box that is the ideal size for holding all of your worries and frustrations overnight while you sleep. Look for it now and when you find it, put it on your nightstand. This is where you'll store all your troubles, crises, frustrations, debts and doubts for safekeeping overnight. Keep it close-by (Lord knows how we cherish our problems), but far enough away to not bother you while you sleep— stress-free. Maybe if you decorate it, you might attract an angel or an elf who wants to help solve your problems overnight.

MAKE FRIENDS WITH ELVES AND ANGELS

Make a friend of that elf, angel or "spirit" who is watching over you, the patient and your problems. Say "hi" on occasion during the day. Ask for help or a blessing as you're sliding into dreamland at night. Important: If you find comfort in prayers, say them before you begin your nighttime progressive relaxation countdown.

MOTIVATION MEDITATIONS

There are oodles of daily meditation books available these days. If you have a favorite, please continue to read it. I still read my favorites.

However, the motivation meditations at the end of the chapter are different from most. They reflect the mental gymnastics I had to exercise when I realized that relieving the stress of caregiving and brain rehabilitation was now a major part of my life. As you know, I didn't want to climb this mountain. But if I continued to dread my days and my new life's work, I'd soon lose my mind, spirit, and eventually, my health, to the stress.

Personally, I'm a doodler by nature. Anytime I participate in a business meeting, my notebook is festooned with pencil sketches of optical illusions, birch trees (I guess I like to draw peeling bark), and profiles of (don't laugh) the Beatles—with and without moustaches. Sometimes my coworkers ask if I'm bored with the meeting. Not true. Somehow, someway, doodling helps me focus on the situation or problem we're discussing. The rhythm of drawing helps me relax. Most importantly, in this altered state, the door to my subconscious mind is opened. That's where ideas flow and my mind makes intuitive connections that produce creative solutions to the problems and challenges at hand.

Some folks can arrive at the same mental state through knitting, gardening, baking, beading or whittling, etc. That's good. But like doodling, these repetitive, creative crafting skills are not usually shared by both caregiver and patient.

However, coloring with crayons, pencils or markers is a crafting skill we all know and practiced for years. As you may remember from your childhood school days, you and your fellow classmates were never quieter, more engaged or better behaved than during coloring time in school. Coloring is soothing, relaxing and a natural stress reliever in the stroke/brain injury healing environment.

Though the following motivational meditation coloring projects are primarily designed for the caregiver, we can easily make them work simultaneously as therapy for the patient. While the caregiver can use the time to quickly manage stress and set the stage for a creative, motivated approach to living the day, the patient might use the exercise for relearning how to focus, pay attention to the moment or practice hand-eye coordination. It is the spirit of "we will get better together" in action. Thus the coloring project becomes a daily multifaceted exercise where caregiver and patient can "hold hands", motivationally-speaking, and begin the day on common ground. After fifteen minutes of coloring and meditating together, they can proceed with the day and better meet the physical/mental/emotional challenges it holds for both of them.

We've talked a lot about how important it is for the patient to feel satisfaction and pride in accomplishing the daily routine. Well, so it is for the caregiver, too, especially on an emotional level. That's why these motivational meditations are divided into morning and evening exercises, so you can celebrate your daily progress. Try it for 21 days. See if taking these small steps toward controlling stress, becoming motivated and reinforcing positive behaviors makes you feel more relaxed, more in control and just plain healthier—physically, mentally and emotionally.

By the way, large versions of each coloring page can be found on my web site (Eurekamaster.com). Just click and print one or two copies of each one.

A FINAL THOUGHT

This is not logical.

You are absolutely right. This is not logical—it is emotional.

Perhaps you're thinking you don't have time for imagination exercises right now. That's what I thought. However, we are dealing with emotions—not logic. It's emotions that will wreak havoc with your physical and mental health. I'm sure your logic's fine. (If not, contact a scientist for more information.) However, stress is born of emotions gone wild. We have to battle it on its terms—no matter how illogical that appears.

A word of caution: don't try this alone. Ask someone for daily support as you implement and customize the Eureka! strategy in your daily routines. You can talk to each other—caregiver to caregiver—via the message board at Eurekamaster.com. You can also contact me via that message board or directly. You'll see when you visit my Web site.

Now, it's time for the daily meditations. Take three deep breaths. We are on our way to getting better together.

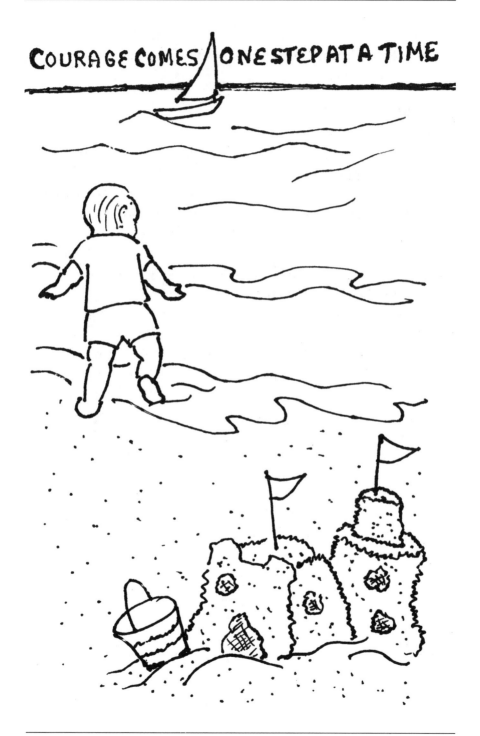

COURAGE COMES ONE STEP AT A TIME

Courage comes one step at a time.

Morning Motivation: Color Yourself Courageous

Lots of people agree that being a caregiver takes more than a little courage. There are days when crises come from the world around us. Other days, the trouble starts inside our heads. For some, the isolation becomes so comfortable, it takes courage to go outside for a walk. Others fear paying the bills or trying to bargain with the insurance/medical establishment. Whatever your personal battle-ground, respect any and all courageous actions you take today.

Today's Goals:
For Me _____
For the Patient _____
For Us_____

Evening Revelation: I caught a glimpse of my courage today. I overcame one of my fears by taking a few steps in the right direction. I would not call myself courageous – or would I? I'm learning to respect my own acts of courage.

Positive Things That Happened Today (To Me, To Us):

_____

_____

_____

Gratitude-With-A-Twist-List: Here are the mini-miracles I experienced today. I was not controlling—these were gifts from the heavens. For this, I am grateful.

_____

_____

_____

_____

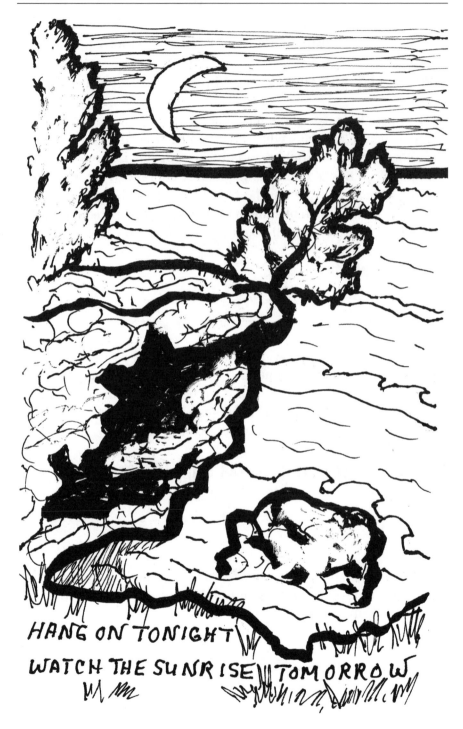

HANG ON TONIGHT
WATCH THE SUNRISE TOMORROW

Hang on tonight. Watch the sunrise tomorrow.

Morning Motivation: Color Yourself Tenacious

Can't move forward today? Sometimes just hanging on is a feat. So, hang on for another hour, another day, another night. Meanwhile, see if life doesn't deliver a little miracle or two while you persist in hanging on and hoping. Sometimes time can be our best friend; but we have to be patient and vigilant, so we can learn why.

Today's Goals:

For Me _____

For the Patient _____

For Us_____

Evening Revelation: Hour by hour, all I could do was hang on. I'm so glad I did, because now I know I can survive without losing hope for positive progress tomorrow.

Positive Things That Happened Today (To Me, To Us):

_____

_____

_____

Gratitude-With-A-Twist-List: Here are the mini-miracles I experienced today. I was not controlling—these were gifts from the heavens. For this, I am grateful.

_____

_____

_____

_____

_____

_____

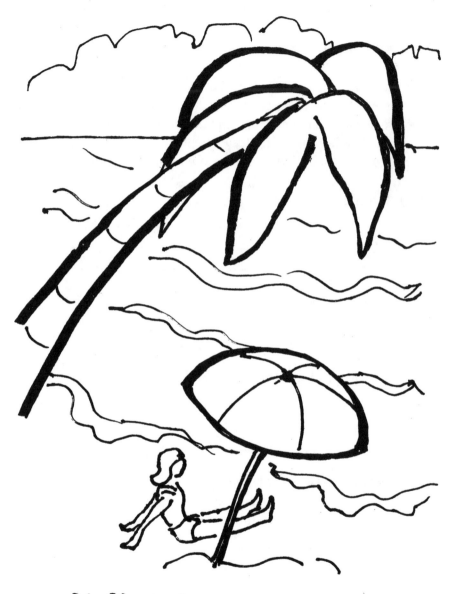

ALWAYS REMEMBER
HOW THE SUNSHINE FEELS

Always remember how the sunshine feels.

Morning Motivation: Color Yourself Relaxed

One . . . breathe in. Two . . . exhale your frustrations. Three . . . breathe in. Four . . . exhale your worries. Five . . . breathe in. Six . . . exhale your stress. If your problems haven't gone away yet, do it again. Then imagine basking in the summer sun on a sandy beach. Wiggle those toes; fingers, too. Stretch your neck. Feel the warm sun soothing your neck, your back. Ah-h-h. Practice frequently until you understand why.

Today's Goals:

For Me _____

For the Patient _____

For Us_____

Evening Revelation: I practiced relaxation today. I had to constantly remind myself to try it. (That's a measure of how much stress I've stuffed into my poor little body.) Perhaps tomorrow I won't have to work so hard at relaxing. I'll do it just for fun—and relaxation, of course.

Positive Things That Happened Today (To Me, To Us):

_____

_____

_____

Gratitude-With-A-Twist-List: Here are the mini-miracles I experienced today. I was not controlling—these were gifts from the heavens. For this, I am grateful.

_____

_____

_____

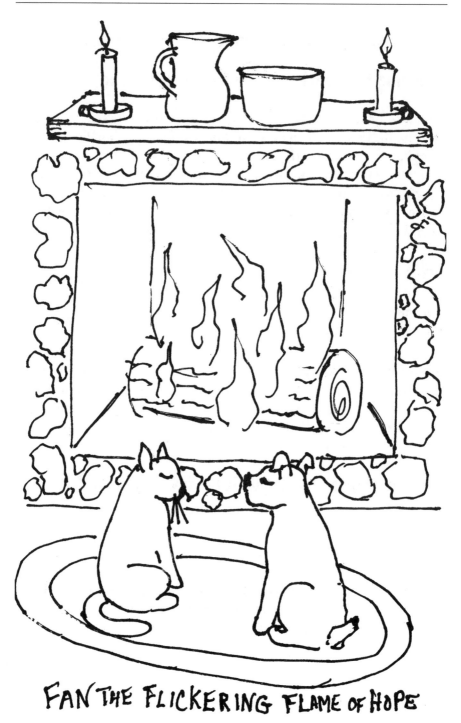

FAN THE FLICKERING FLAME OF HOPE

Fan the flickering flame of hope.

Morning Motivation: Color Yourself Hopeful

One day I heard myself say to somebody, "I have no hope for Eve's full recovery." In retrospect, I now know those words were spoken in anger and fear, just in case God and the angels were listening. In truth, Eve's recovery had little to do with how much I hoped for it. That made me feel powerless and angry. However, I did have a tee-nie-tiny bit of hope that I could make our home a more positive healing environment, in case Eve's brain wanted to get well. My only job was to fan the fire of hope and act on it. It was up to Eve and the heavens to use my efforts as they saw fit.

Today's Goals:
For Me _____
For the Patient _____
For Us_____

Evening Revelation: After reading this morning's meditation, I hoped I could make a better contribution to our recovery environment. Surprise! I acted on that feeling and got what I hoped for. Tonight I can relax in front of the fireplace knowing that I am a better caregiver than I was this morning.

Positive Things That Happened Today (To Me, To Us):

_____

_____

_____

Gratitude-With-A-Twist-List: Here are the mini-miracles I experienced today. I was not controlling—these were gifts from the heavens. For this, I am grateful.

_____

_____

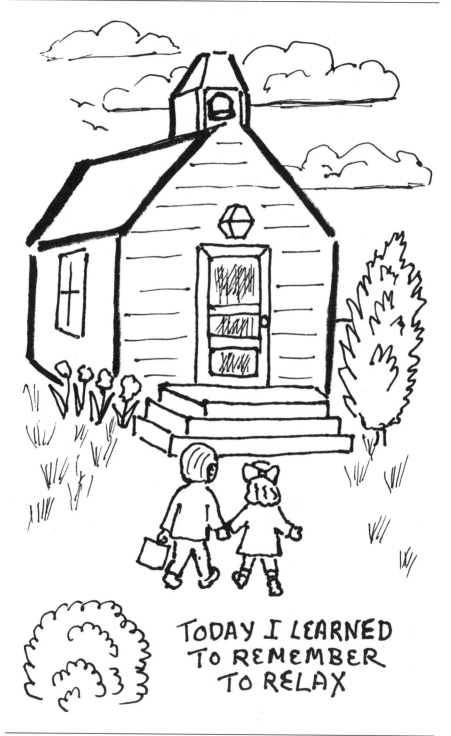

Today I learned to remember to relax.

Morning Motivation: Color Yourself Teachable

It's nigh impossible to learn anything new when we are anxious or stressed. In order to learn how to handle caregiving, we must first relax. Coloring can help us remember how relaxation feels. Remember, there is nothing new except what is forgotten.

Today's Goals:

For Me _____

For the Patient _____

For Us_____

Evening Revelation: I thought about being teachable versus thinking I had all the answers. Good thing. Today I learned something "old" I had almost forgotten: I learned how relaxing coloring can be.

Positive Things That Happened Today (To Me, To Us):

_____

_____

_____

Gratitude-With-A-Twist-List: Here are the mini-miracles I experienced today. I was not controlling—these were gifts from the heavens. For this, I am grateful.

_____

_____

_____

_____

_____

_____

_____

WHY CHASE IT?
INSPIRATION WILL COME TO YOU

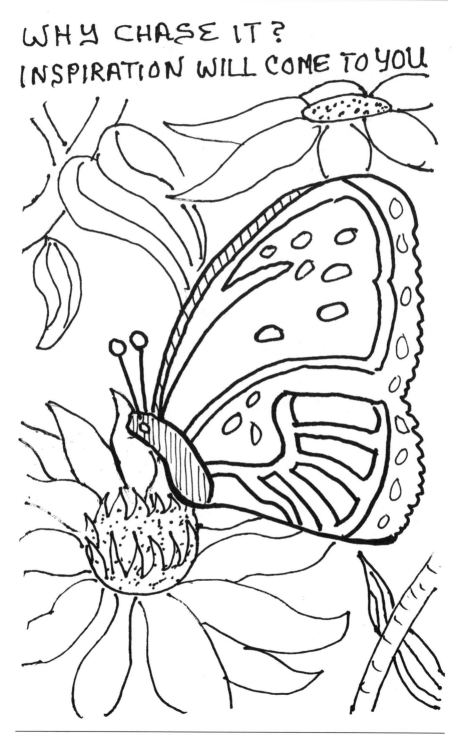

Why chase it? Inspiration will come to you.

Morning Motivation: Color Yourself Inspired

Way back when I was a kid, one of my school friends gave me a gift. It was an inexpensive little plaque with a Nathaniel Hawthorne quote. I was too young to understand the quote—but not too young to memorize it. "Happiness is as a butterfly, which when pursued is always beyond our grasp. But if one sits quietly, it will alight upon a shoulder." Interestingly, it's also true for inspiration.

Today's Goals:

For Me _____

For the Patient _____

For Us_____

Evening Revelation: I admit it. I still chase butterflies (with my camera, of course). It never fails. Whenever I stop to catch my breath, that's when a butterfly alights on a flower right in front of me. If only I would patiently watch and wait for that flutter of inspiration to come to me, I wouldn't have to run around in circles.

Positive Things That Happened Today (To Me, To Us):

_____

_____

_____

Gratitude-With-A-Twist-List: Here are the mini-miracles I experienced today. I was not controlling—these were gifts from the heavens. For this, I am grateful.

_____

_____

_____

_____

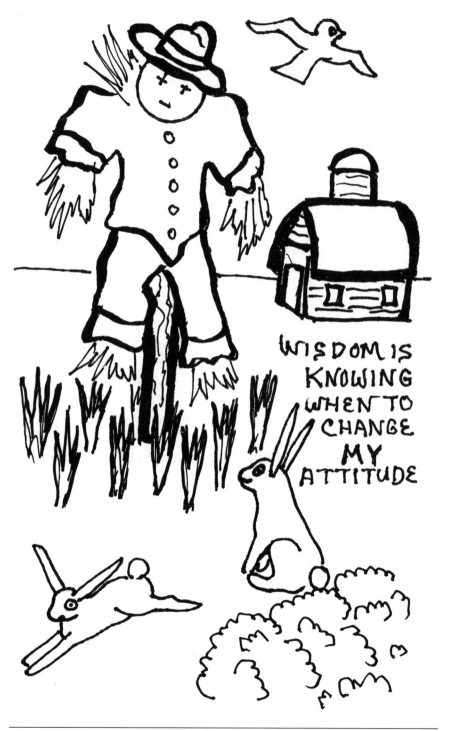

WISDOM IS KNOWING WHEN TO CHANGE MY ATTITUDE

Wisdom is knowing when to change my attitude.

Morning Motivation: Color Yourself Wise

Ordinary people can be smart; but wisdom is reserved for judges, philosophers, theologians and really old people. That's what I thought, until I said the Serenity Prayer for the umpteenth time. The prayer is: God, Grant me the serenity to accept the things I cannot change; the courage to change the things I can; and the wisdom to know the difference. After dealing with brain healing for this long, I believe I'm beginning to know the difference. I can't change the patient; I can only change me.

Today's Goals:

For Me _____

For the Patient _____

For Us_____

Evening Revelation: The more I work on changing myself to accept life on life's terms, the wiser I become. Now that I know that, I'm working on accepting my rate of change.

Positive Things That Happened Today (To Me, To Us):

_____

_____

_____

Gratitude-With-A-Twist-List: Here are the mini-miracles I experienced today. I was not controlling—these were gifts from the heavens. For this, I am grateful.

_____

_____

_____

_____

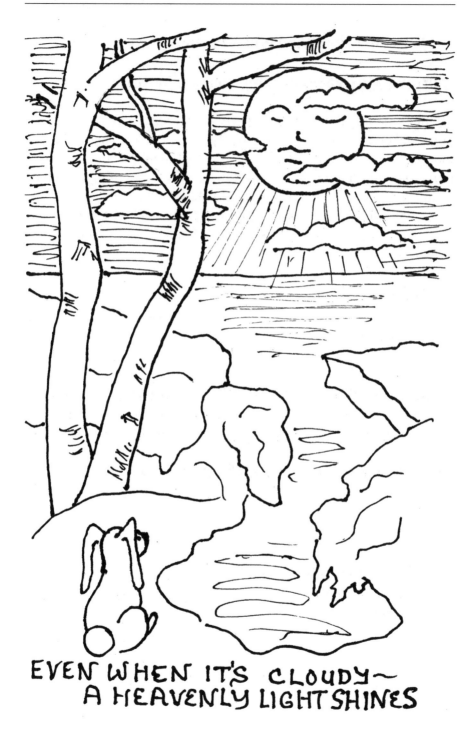

EVEN WHEN IT'S CLOUDY~
A HEAVENLY LIGHT SHINES

Even when it's cloudy, a heavenly light shines.

Morning Motivation: Color Yourself Cared For

When the night is dark and lonely, there's comfort in knowing someone cares. No one does, you say? Might the problem be that you are dictating how they show it? Think again. Think about all the weird, wonderful and unique ways your family, friends and neighbors show they care. See? They do care. But if I need more, then it's up to me to join a local or online support group. I can investigate my options today.

Today's Goals:
For Me _____
For the Patient _____
For Us_____

Evening Revelation: I thought about how my friends and family have tried to show they care. Some were awesome, others so-so; and a few tickled me with their attempts. But care they did, to the best of their abilities. What didn't work for me was expecting folks to care the way I wanted them to care. So today I took steps to join a group. Tomorrow, I'll take more.

Positive Things That Happened Today (To Me, To Us):

_____

_____

_____

Gratitude-With-A-Twist-List: Here are the mini-miracles I experienced today. I was not controlling—these were gifts from the heavens. For this, I am grateful.

_____

_____

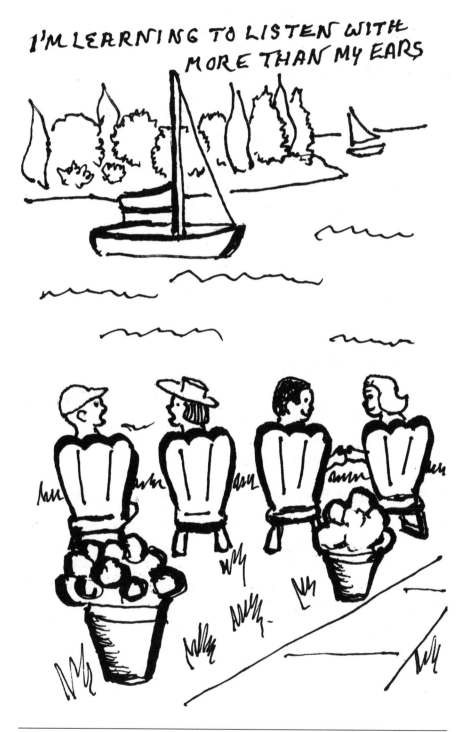

I'm learning to listen with more than my ears.

Morning Motivation: Color Yourself a Communicator

When talking to the patient these days, I realize how many of our pre-aneurysm conversations were jibber-jabber. Hour upon hour was filled with mindless chitchat. Now I devote much more time to purposeful two-way communication. I'm more in tune with listening. Now I really do care about what the patient says, and how, and why. At long last, we are communicating.

Today's Goals:
For Me _____

For the Patient _____

For Us_____

Evening Revelation: I made the effort today to do more listening and less talking. I'm learning to listen with my eyes as well as my ears. I'm learning to "feel" the patient's message. Nowadays, we communicate more than we ever did before.

Positive Things That Happened Today (To Me, To Us):

_____

_____

_____

Gratitude-With-A-Twist-List: Here are the mini-miracles I experienced today. I was not controlling—these were gifts from the heavens. It'll be a fine day indeed when I run out of lines and need to record more miracles in the margins of the page

_____

_____

_____

_____

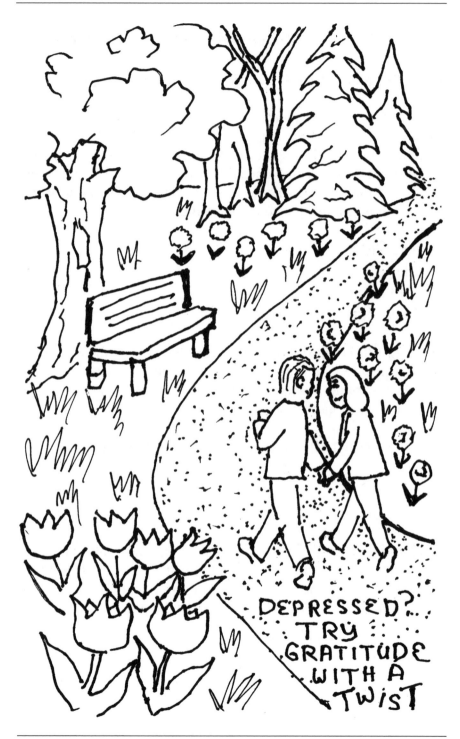

Depressed? Try gratitude with a twist.

Morning Motivation: Color Yourself Grateful

Interestingly, I've never felt depressed and grateful at the same time. But sometimes I've awakened with a cloud hovering over my head. It used to be hard work to think myself out of my depression. One day I discovered an incredibly easy, quick fix. I create an instant miracle. All I do is close my eyes wherever I am (except driving a car) and try to negotiate the terrain. I can't travel ten feet without bumping into a wall. Ouch! Walking around the front yard is downright scary. But a minute of walking blind does the trick. I am so very grateful when I open my eyes. Thank God, I can see.

Today's Goals:

For Me _____

For the Patient _____

For Us_____

Evening Revelation: Nothing flips my day around faster than switching to an attitude of gratitude. I'm even learning to be grateful for my problems. So many of them come into my life bearing gifts.

Positive Things That Happened Today (To Me, To Us):

_____

_____

_____

Gratitude-With-A-Twist-List: Here are the mini-miracles I experienced today. I was not controlling—these were gifts from the heavens. For this, I am grateful.

_____

_____

_____

WHEN ALL ELSE FAILS...

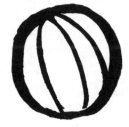

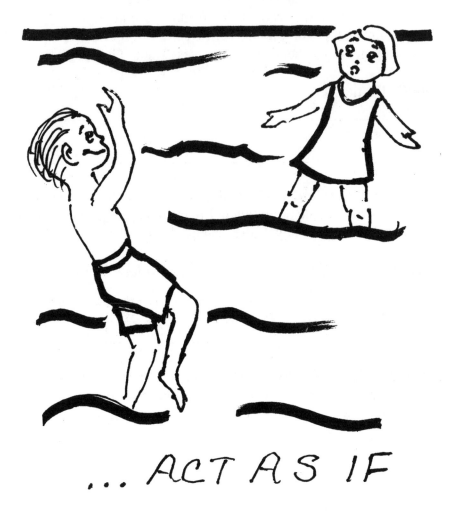

... ACT AS IF

When all else fails, act as if.

Morning Motivation: Color Yourself Enthusiastic

I feel so depleted and depressed this morning. I tried, but I can't "act as if" I am feeling enthusiastic. No, I am not going to try again." So there, I win, don't I? Well, maybe not.

Today's Goals:
For Me _____

For the Patient _____

For Us_____

Evening Revelation: I get it! If I'm willing to try to "act as if" I'm enthusiastic, eventually it will kick in. It works like magic. And it makes life so much easier. That's a lot of payback for a little bit of trying.

Positive Things That Happened Today (To Me, To Us):

_____

_____

_____

Gratitude-With-A-Twist-List: Here are the mini-miracles I experienced today. I was not controlling—these were gifts from the heavens. For this, I am grateful.

_____

_____

_____

_____

_____

_____

_____

_____

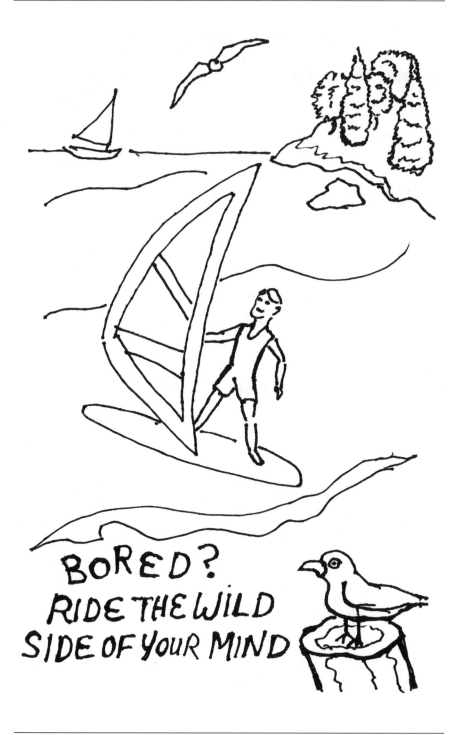

Bored? Ride the "wild" side of your mind.

Morning Motivation: Color Yourself Adventurous

No, you don't have to fly over the waves on a tiny surfboard. But you can do something—anything—differently. Finding adventure is as easy as visiting the public library. Pick out a movie, CD or book you'd never, ever normally choose. Surprise yourself with how daring you really are. Adventure awaits you tonight.

Today's Goals:

For Me _____

For the Patient _____

For Us_____

Evening Revelation: Wow! That library trip was as much fun as riding the wild surf—easier, too. I brought home all sorts of intriguing CDs, DVDs and books. I'm exploring my wild side tonight.

Positive Things That Happened Today (To Me, To Us):

_____

_____

_____

Gratitude-With-A-Twist-List: Here are the mini-miracles I experienced today. I was not controlling—these were gifts from the heavens. It'll be a fine day indeed when I run out of lines and need to record more miracles in the margins of the page.

_____

_____

_____

_____

_____

_____

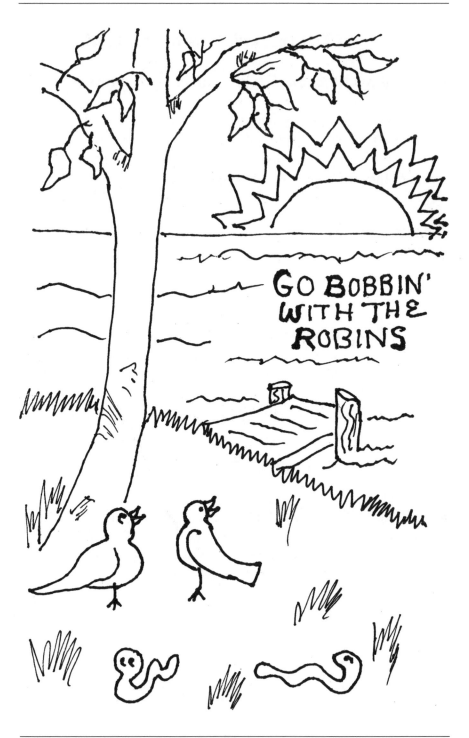

Feeling blah? Go bobbin' with the robins.

Morning Motivation: Color Yourself Energized

After breakfast, step outside. Breathe in the energy of a brand-new day. Is the air warm and inviting? Chilly and invigorating? Lush with rain? Mellowed by snow? Crystal-clear with cold? Hot and soothing? Take whatever energy you need from whatever nature offers. It's your first gift of the day. Take one deep breath now . . . and then take some more. The energy is free. So's the robin's cheery song.

Today's Goals:

For Me _____

For the Patient _____

For Us_____

Evening Revelation: How quickly the blahs went away when I took time to breathe in the energy of the day. With a couple of gulps of fresh air, nature delivered the tonic I needed to embrace the day's challenges.

Positive Things That Happened Today (To Me, To Us):

_____

_____

_____

Gratitude-With-A-Twist-List: Here are the mini-miracles I experienced today. I was not controlling—these were gifts from the heavens. For this, I am grateful.

_____

_____

_____

_____

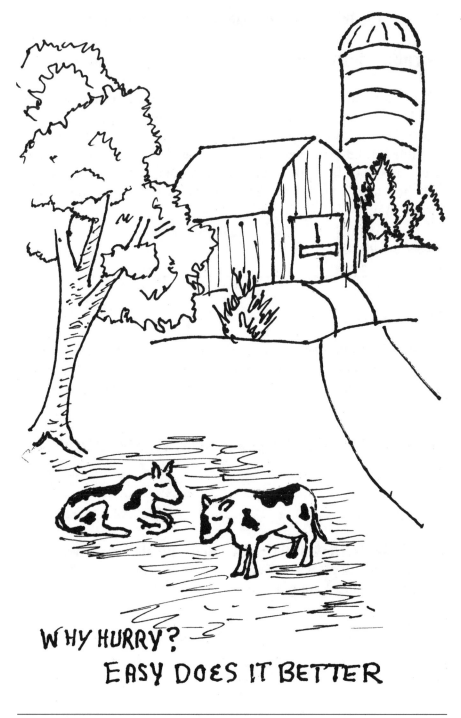

WHY HURRY?
EASY DOES IT BETTER

Why hurry? Easy does it better.

Morning Motivation: Color Yourself Patient

S-l-o-w down. Mosey over to that shady rest area in your mind. Take your time coloring this picture. The rewards come when you chew on things slowly. Pace yourself to color half of the picture in the morning, the rest in the evening. Perhaps you'll see something you've been missing in your race to solve your problems.

Today's Goals:

For Me _____

For the Patient _____

For Us_____

Evening Revelation: S-l-o-w-i-n-g down helps us pay attention to the dynamics of the problems we may have encountered today. Slowly chewing on a challenge helps. It is always best to take problem-solving slowly so the subconscious mind has a chance to help. Like milk, all good things take time.

Positive Things That Happened Today (To Me, To Us):

_____

_____

_____

Gratitude-With-A-Twist-List: Here are the mini-miracles I experienced today. I was not controlling—these were gifts from the heavens. For this, I am grateful.

_____

_____

_____

_____

_____

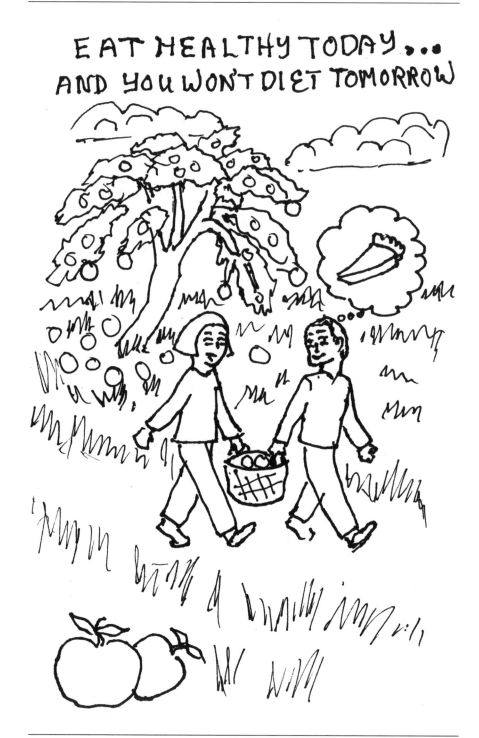

Eat healthy today and you won't diet tomorrow.

Morning Motivation: Color Yourself Healthier

Dieting is such a drag. It's much easier to balance a meal, hold the salt, minimize sugar and drink more water. Give it a try tonight. Balance meals with the five food groups: dairy, vegetables, fruit, meat—and dessert. Then put dieting on your to-do list next to "plan a cruise".

Today's Goals:

For Me _____

For the Patient _____

For Us_____

Evening Revelation: Dessert? That's not a food group. No; but it can be a reward for the patient and you. Don't obsess about eating too many sweets. When you realize their huge potential as rewards, you'll naturally want to limit them for special occasions. As for daily desserts, we like canned pineapple and slivered almonds mixed into vanilla yogurt. How deliciously healthy can you get?

Positive Things That Happened Today (To Me, To Us):

_____

_____

_____

Gratitude-With-A-Twist-List: Here are the mini-miracles I experienced today. I was not controlling—these were gifts from the heavens. For this, I am grateful.

_____

_____

_____

_____

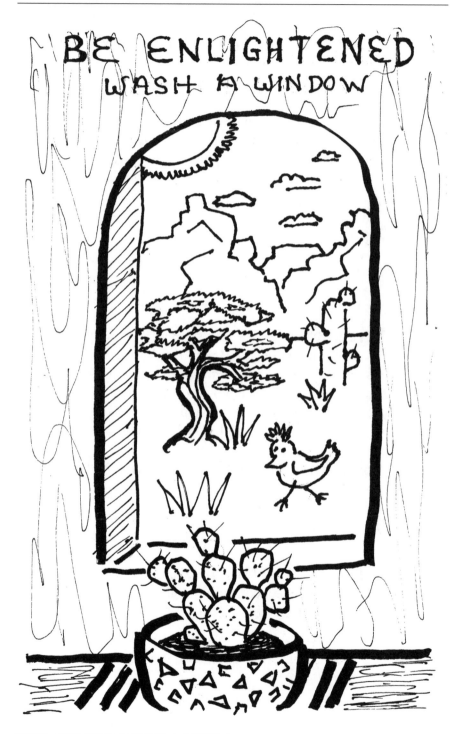

Be enlightened. Wash a window.

Morning Motivation: Color Yourself Enlightened

Is your mind spinning? Do you spend hours googling for answers? I've been there. Stuck in a chair, staring out a window, wondering if anything I could do would make any difference. Well, there is something you and I can do. We can get a bottle of spray and a paper towel and clean that dirty window. Then we can do another one. Soon we'll feel enlightened—and all sorts of good ideas will come to us.

Today's Goals:

For Me _____

For the Patient _____

For Us_____

Evening Revelation: Boy, oh boy, washing windows makes me feel so much better than contemplating my bellybutton. From now on, whenever I'm "spinning", I'll just take an action. Any action is better than none. When my windows are clean, the world seems so much brighter—and I feel enlightened.

Positive Things That Happened Today (To Me, To Us):

_____

_____

_____

Gratitude-With-A-Twist-List: Here are the mini-miracles I experienced today. I was not controlling—these were gifts from the heavens. For this, I am grateful.

_____

_____

_____

_____

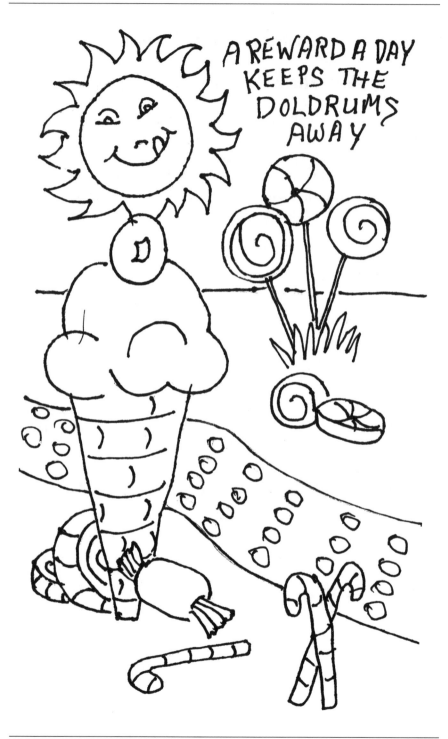

A reward a day keeps the doldrums away.

Morning Motivation: Color Yourself Motivated

Never underestimate the allure of a sweet treat to power us through a ho-hum day. Not just candy. We can also treat ourselves to a TV show, computer game, crossword puzzle or book. If we limit our indulgences throughout the week, then these little motivations become rewards to anticipate.

Today's Goals:

For Me _____

For the Patient _____

For Us_____

Evening Revelation: We can manipulate ourselves with little motivations that make days more interesting and (dare I say it) fun. There's no (healthy) excuse for not having a bit of fun every day.

Positive Things That Happened Today (To Me, To Us):

_____

_____

_____

Gratitude-With-A-Twist-List: Here are the mini-miracles I experienced today. I was not controlling—these were gifts from the heavens. For this, I am grateful.

_____

_____

_____

_____

_____

_____

_____

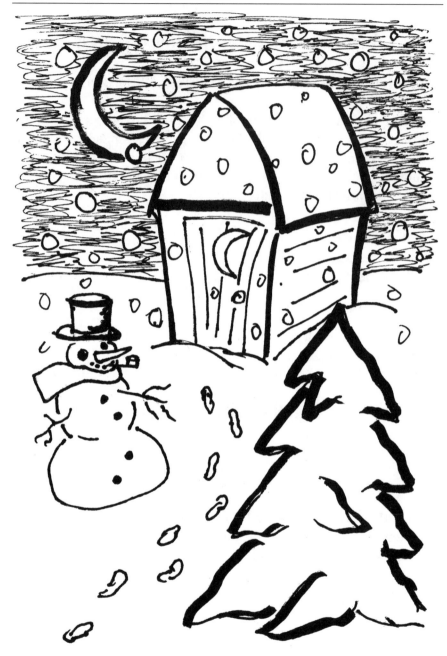

CHOOSE TO BE HAPPY

Take a shortcut to good health. Choose to be happy.

Morning Motivation: Color Yourself Happy

Me, happy? You've got to be kidding. Look at the mess we're in. I can't possibly be happy, until we are well again. That's absolutely correct. No one can be happy if one chooses not to be happy until the other person changes for the better. But that's how I felt, until I realized how ludicrous my logic was. Even with our misfortunes, we still had our house, food on the table, winter jackets—and indoor plumbing. (If nothing else, I could be very happy about the comforts of a warm bathroom on a frigid night.)

Today's Goals:
For Me _____

For the Patient _____

For Us_____

Evening Revelation: I realize now that I have choices. One choice is to be a relaxed and healthy caregiver. Today I can choose to act as if I'm happy. That's as easy as deciding if I should trade in our lovely toilet for an outhouse.

Positive Things That Happened Today (To Me, To Us):

_____

_____

_____

Gratitude-With-A-Twist-List: Here are the mini-miracles I experienced today. I was not controlling—these were gifts from the heavens. For this, I am grateful.

_____

_____

_____

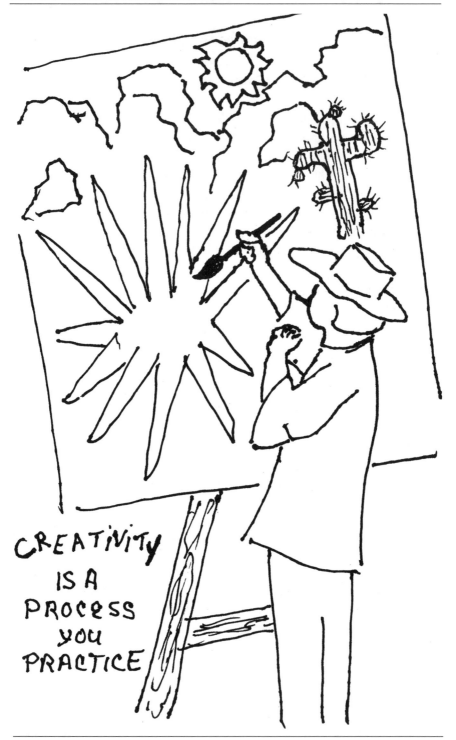

CREATIVITY IS A PROCESS YOU PRACTICE

Creativity is a process you practice.

Morning Motivation: Color Yourself Creative

As I began creatively coloring this Arizona high desert picture, my imagination took me away from the snowy Midwest. For a few moments I was free to hike this pretty trail in sunny Red Rock Country. The more I exercise the power of creativity, the better I can express it.

Today's Goals:
For Me _____

For the Patient _____

For Us_____

Evening Revelation: Today I practiced creativity. For the moment, I am "acting as if" I am creative. However, I believe that if I keep practicing the process, I too will feel the magic of creativity. I'll know it when I feel the spark.

Positive Things That Happened Today (To Me, To Us):

_____

_____

_____

Gratitude-With-A-Twist-List: Here are the mini-miracles I experienced today. I was not controlling—these were gifts from the heavens. For this, I am grateful.

_____

_____

_____

_____

_____

_____

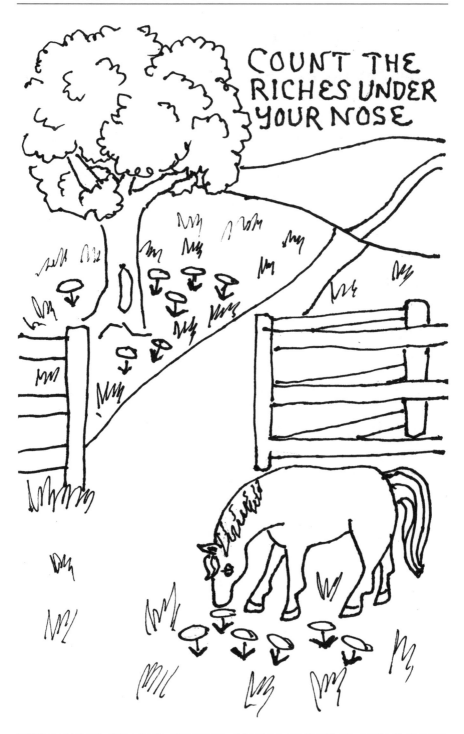

Count the Riches Under Your Nose.

Morning Motivation: Color Yourself Content

If I am feeling discontented with my lot in life, I check my expectations level first. Then I focus on appreciating what I have—and have not—been given for my "life" test. Like me, maybe you have a few friends who are having a harder time than we are. Um, maybe we could give them a supportive call this evening?

Today's Goals:

For Me _____

For the Patient _____

For Us_____

Evening Revelation: I often recite this little prayer: Dear God: Thank You for all You have given me, all You have taken from me, and all You have left me. That's one motivational sentence that nudges me to be grateful that God didn't give me what I deserved.

Positive Things That Happened Today (To Me, To Us):

_____

_____

_____

Gratitude-With-A-Twist-List: Here are the mini-miracles I experienced today. I was not controlling—these were gifts from the heavens. For this, I am grateful.

_____

_____

_____

_____

_____

_____

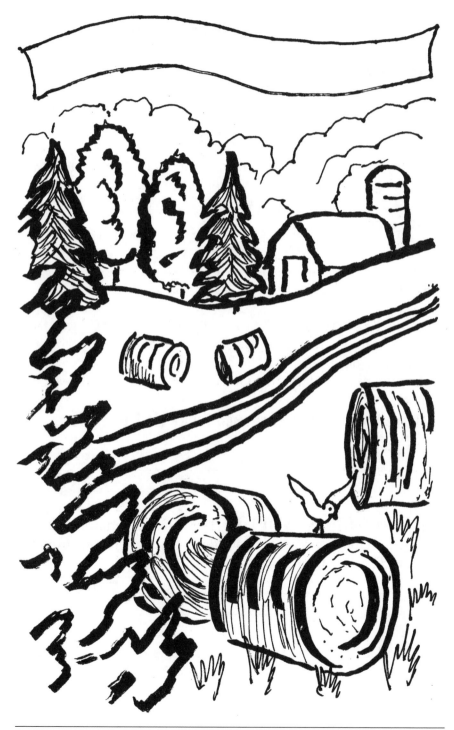

EUREKA! COLORING ADVENTURES AT HOME

Now, here is the coloring motivation meditation for your weekly Eureka! activity. The featured coloring project is one of my favorite art subjects, hay bales. If you live in the Midwest, this is a familiar farmland sight in autumn.

So, what is the unique selling point of this seemingly blah bale of hay? Interestingly, it is one of the most-painted subjects in the world of art. That famous Impressionist painter, Claude Monet, painted oodles of hay bale pictures. Monet immortalized these "lumps of dried grass" by portraying them in all sorts of weather, at different times of day and different seasons of the year. He transformed an ordinary, everyday, blah object into great works of art that are worth millions of dollars, and showcased in museums around the world.

My point is that outside every window is a multi-million dollar "hay bale" painting waiting to happen. When you pause during your coloring project, take a peek outside and search for your own mesmerizing hay bale. Yes, you do have one. Can you see a mountain or a lake that changes hour by hour? How about that old oak tree? Do different birds visit it seasonally? Do the leaves change colors? How about that cactus? Is it ready to bloom?

If all else fails, look at the sky. Is it a warm, summery azure-blue? A crispy, cool minty-blue? An evening shade of indigo? What color are the clouds and what shape are they in? Where's the sun? Is there a daytime moon?

You too can immortalize the ordinary for your patient and create Eureka! memories with your play-by-play.

Here's a little help. You can begin by jotting down a ten-word action phrase, such as "Every day in every way we are getting better together." or "Soon we will be driving country roads together again." This is your own personal slogan for the day. Write that phrase in the "slogan box "at the top of the hay bale picture.

As you begin coloring together, keep the conversation rolling by talking about your memories of visits to the farm, car rides over country roads, favorite autumn festivities such as apple picking, pumpkin hunting, burning leaves and jumping in haystacks. Or perhaps you love art, too, and have fond memories of exhibitions that featured Monet's not-so-ordinary hay bale paintings.

It's all in how you perceive—and communicate—the scents, sights and sensual delights and those powerful emotions of the moment. It's Eureka!—and you are making it happen your way today.

24

Ah, Sweet Success

By now you know how this 21-day stress-reduction program is working for you. Keep trying. I hope you've personalized this program with your favorite methods for relaxing and developing intuition.

On the caregiving front, I hope you have a clearer view of how to progress from hourly projects to a daily routine, punctuated with Eureka! play hours that are challenging, creative and interesting for both of you. Perhaps you've even tried a few Eureka! activities. As with anything creative, the more you do it, the more Eureka! ideas you will be blessed with by that great creative source in the sky.

Meanwhile, you'll be busy organizing your daily support system. Remember, you can always ask me for support. I'm available most every day at www.Eurekamaster.com. Why? I realize that my own strength for caregiving comes from sharing whatever helpful ideas or actions I have experienced.

This attitude and approach can work for you, too. Whether you are asking for help or giving it, visit my Web site. See (and feel) how and why sharing our caregiving experiences can help all of us. Remember that most of us will be on this journey for the rest of our lives. Let's travel together.

Afterword

Remember all the times I've told you we caregivers need a support network. Well, the following letter is from one of my best supporters, Fannie Tsang from Hong Kong, China. Fannie and I met via e-mail. She wrote me several months ago after she read my first book "Brain, Heal Thyself."

Fannie is the caregiver for her beloved husband, Patrick, age 40, who survived a massive stroke in December, 2008. Now, ten months later, he is recovering in a rehabilitation hospital in Hong Kong, working to restore his paralyzed right side and vocal chords. He's making progress. The going is steady but slow.

I asked Fannie if she would read the manuscript for "Eureka!" and give me her reaction. English is Fannie's second language, but I think her letter needs minimal editing. As brain caregivers, we are always practicing our intuition skills. Following is a great opportunity for all of us to listen with our hearts to Fannie's experience, her highs and lows and her great love for Patrick, as well as her hopes for their future.

Dear Madonna,

Since my Patrick's stroke several months ago, I have been reading everything I can on the subject.

I have an entire bookshelf devoted to stroke patient memoirs, many books describing physical, occupational and speech therapy techniques and lots of "how-to" books on the basics of daily caregiving.

But there's only one book on that shelf that helps both patient and the caregiver, too, get well by fortifying the emotional and spiritual bond between both of them. That book is "Eureka!" and I just agree with every word of it.

There's an ancient Chinese saying that literally translates: "When two hearts combine, they can cut through gold." It brings to mind a visualization of two medieval warriors grabbing one sword and together piercing the armor of their fierce opponent. Neither one has the strength to win the battle alone; but together they can do and beat anything.

This can totally apply to caregiving. Fortunately, most of the caregivers and patients already have that relationship where two hearts are combined. Good friends like Eve and you, spouses like Patrick and I, parents and children or vice-versa, all have combined their hearts to help in this recovery.

But the battle is every day. Although it is a challenge; it can be fun, too. I truly love the phrase: "We will get better together." To me, it means that on the long road to recovery, there's no hierarchy. There's no teacher or student, no mother and daughter, no husband and wife. There's just two uncompromised souls melted together, trying to find their way out by supporting and improving each other.

The longer I take care of Patrick, the more I realize that he is helping me to grow as well.

Before his stroke, I wasn't a strong woman at all—not even close. I was the kind of woman who hides behind her husband's back. I didn't cook (still don't), or take care of the bills, the mortgage or even my tax. They were all Patrick's matters.

So you can imagine how panicked I was when Patrick had the stroke. If worry was a black hole, I was at the bottom of it. But I got a hold of myself. Despite tears and fears, with lots of trials and errors, I have become a much better woman today. Everyone who knew us is totally surprised at how strong and mature I've become.

One thing I am sure of is that God changed me through Patrick's stroke. Somehow I felt that I was the one God wanted to learn the lesson, not Patrick. Without God's power, I might still be crying and complaining in the black hole.

You see, Patrick did help me to grow more mature and to get better. And with that maturity and a finer me, I can help him to recover from the stroke. This is a yin-yang relationship. One alone cannot live without the other. Together they complete each other. Our love has grown stronger than ever. Our relationship is better than it has been in 20 years. Isn't it ironic? We grew better through the darkest time of our lives. I'm so different from the person I was ten months ago. I'm more gentle, caring and, most of all, grateful. Like the book says, I've become exactly the kind of caregiver Patrick needs at this moment.

I also so agreed with the subconscious healing approach, even if there's no scientific proof of that realm. I had tried it on Patrick numerous times a few months back when he was in and out of a comatose state (just like Eve).

I'll give you an example, but first let me tell you a story. It's a little embarrassing. You see, I haven't had a driver's license since my college days in Canada. When I came back to Hong Kong, I just forgot to renew it. Hong Kong is ridiculously small for driving, plus public transportation is convenient and cheap. Anyway, Patrick always did the driving if we needed to travel by car. But whenever we did drive, Patrick always teased me because I would confuse the directions. He'd say I didn't know left from right, which was true, especially when I was in a panic. He always joked that if I ever got a license I'd go to jail the first day for killing someone on the road.

One day while I was chatting with him in the hospital, I had an idea. I said to him, "Since you're in the hospital, maybe I should take the driving test and get a license. What do you think, Patrick?" Since his vocal chords were paralyzed, I had prepared "yes" and "no" signs to communicate with him. I put the signs on his lap. He paused for a little bit, looked at the signs, and positively pushed the "no" one at me.

I was indignant. I said to him, "What are you saying? You just came out of a coma and you're teasing me about my driving?" What's more, he had a little grin on his face. Just like with you and Eve, I could see that the old Patrick was still inside. It was the old Patrick who knew I shouldn't drive and that he should stop me from getting a license.

From that moment on, I knew all we needed to do was unleash that old Patrick. How? I wasn't sure, but I started to chat with him normally. I remind him of things we used to do together, the TV shows or movies we watched. (We loved C.S.I.) I tell him the gossip about people we know. I'm sure it's working because Patrick is getting clearer.

It's like playing treasure hunt. The treasures (the old Patrick and Eve) are spotted. All we need to do is find the right tool to retrieve our treasures. And your book has offered many ideas on how to do that! I pray that it helps a lot more brain trauma sufferers and their families to recover.

Thanks for the book. I was in tears by your honesty, the love you had for Eve, and most of all, the noble hope and faith you had for life and the Higher Power.

Without this love, hope and faith, we would not be writing to each other this day.

Love,
Fannie

Once more, I invite you to visit my Web site, Eurekamaster.com, which I monitor frequently. There you will find emotional support for your endeavors and, of course, motivational billboards to color on your daily journey into creative living and stress-free caregiving.

About the Author

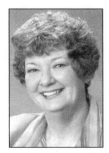

Eureka! Memories and Motivations and *Brain, Heal Thyself* are based on Madonna Siles's experience as the caregiver of her best friend, Eve, the survivor of a near-fatal brain aneurysm, strokes and seizures. Desperate to help her friend, Siles developed a holistic, home rehabilitation plan based on the belief that Eve's subconscious mind would do whatever it takes to help Eve survive.

As the days passed into months, Siles realized that if she didn't start practicing relaxation and stress control for herself, she would be of little help to Eve.

In developing her "home rehabilitation program-for-two", Siles drew from her experience as a practitioner of the 12-step program, her knowledge of subconscious communication techniques, and her experience with motivational techniques gleaned from a career as an advertising communicator. She learned about the subconscious mind's amazing powers, and the various methods to invoke its help in the healing process, while working as a public relations consultant for Lawrence J. Beuret, M.D.

Siles is a Certified Professional Coach specializing in caregiver life coaching. She devotes her free time to artistically expressing the natural beauty of Door County, Wisconsin. She is a graduate of the University of Illinois, Champaign-Urbana, with a B.S. in Communications.

Brain, Heal Thyself

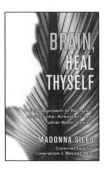

Madonna Siles, C.P.C.
Published June, 2006
Hampton Roads Publishing Company
www.hrpub.com
ISBN 1-57174-476-2

"Brain, Heal Thyself … is one of the most important self-help books on the market … blends memoir and medical insights and will appeal to any caregiver who wants a blend of 'how to' and biography."
Midwest Book Review August, 2006

More Commentary and Resources

When I was beginner caregiver, there was very little on the Internet relating to brain aneurysm rehabilitation. Nowadays, you can find much more if you like to "Google."

You'll find excellent educational information and support links at the American Stroke Association (strokeassociation.org), National Stroke Association (stroke.org), Reeve Foundation (christopherreeve.org) and the numerous state Brain Injury Association web sites (mine is biaw.org). I regularly visit the healthy librarian at happyhealthylonglife.com for tips on taking care of me. Eve is trying out journalafterbraininjury.wordpress.com.

Following are comments about the *Eureka!* book and strategy from web site administrators and authors.

"....as a survivor of a cerebral aneurysm rupture I would hope that every caregiver be given the opportunity to read this book and implement the theories. So often I see that patients who seem to be slow to respond are given up on. Insurance companies are reluctant to pay for continuous therapy. Some patients are lucky they have someone in their life like Madonna Siles, who refused to give up. Maybe the reason that there is little known about the recovery of a patient that survives an aneurysm rupture or an AVM rupture is that this is a new breed. In the past it was basically unheard of for someone to survive such an injury. We are an enigma to the medical professionals and we can be instrumental in teaching them how to treat us and also in the instructions they share with the caregivers. The dedication, the trials and yes the tribulations that Eve and Madonna encountered will be the inspiration for another caregiver and patient!"

Susan Weinholtz, Author of *Time For Uncle Guido*, Administrator—Aneurysm/AVM Support web site (stu.westga.edu/~wmaples)

More Commentary and Resources

"Caregiving is fundamental in determining the progress and quality of life of the patient. If the caregiver does not have goals, or avenues to relieve stress and find enjoyment, this will impact on the patient. *Eureka!* guides the caregiver on how to find their own focus in life. By creating and taking advantage of 'Eureka! Moments', Siles shows that the caregiver and patient can work together and participate in activities and adventures that are enjoyable and motivating, but also help to trigger memories, language and social interaction."

Johan Langfield, Speech and Language Therapist, Founder—icommunicatetherapy.com

(This book is) "compassionate, empathetic, candid, conversational in style, and enlightening for caregiver and survivor alike. Time and again, the author highlights the criticality of 'authentic action' as moving the Eureka process from fiction to fact, from theory into *reality.* The caregiver and survivor will survive and thrive!"

Walter H. Steinlauf, Executive Director, The Stroke Survivors Advocacy Network—strokesurvivorsandcaregivers.ning.com

".... in reading *Eureka!* I found many suggestions that were very possible and applicable to being a parent/caregiver of a teenager with a traumatic brain injury. I, too, identified with many things in my own life that I had to give up. *Eureka!* has changed how I look at my identity and how it relates to this new normal; thus, making my daughter's recovery and rehabilitation a partnership."

Karen "Kasey" Johanson, Parent/TBI Advocate at www.caringbridge.org/visit/kaitlynjohanson

"Madonna has made daily life more interesting for me than it was before my cerebral hemorrhage. I want to help others by contributing to our *Eureka!* web site."

Eve Kasper, Brain Aneurysm Survivor, at eurekamaster.com